10-minute Yoga

10-minute Yoga

100 Personal Programmes for Daily Practice

Donald Butler

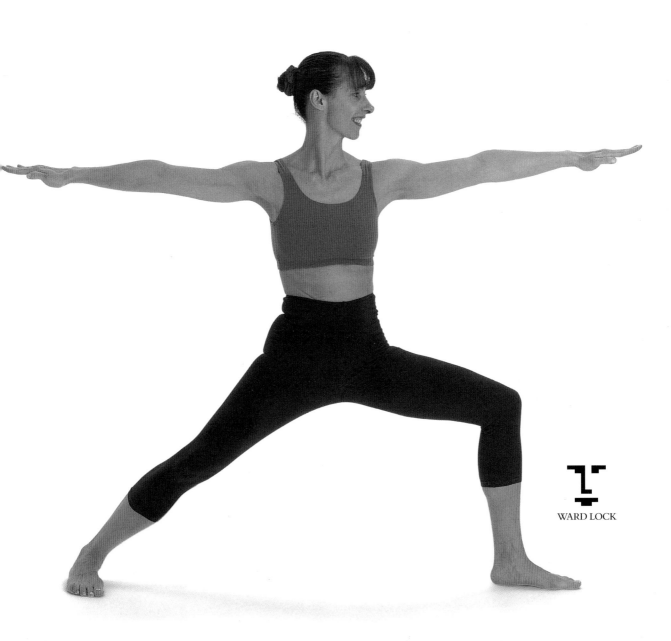

WARD LOCK

A WARD LOCK BOOK

First published in the UK in 1999 by
Ward Lock
Illustrated Division
The Orion Publishing Group
Wellington House
125 Strand
London WC2R 0BB

www.cassell.co.uk

Distributed in the United States by
Sterling Publishing Co., Inc.
387 Park Avenue South
New York NY 10016-8810

British Library Cataloguing-in-Publication Data
A catalogue record for this book is available from
the British Library

ISBN 0-7063-7814-8

Photography by Steve Shott
Designed by Yvonne Dedman

Printed by Wing King Tong Co., Hong Kong

The author and publishers would
like to thank the following models:
Steve Austen
Roger King
Zoë Knott
Jacqueline Purnell

Thanks are also due to Espree Leisure Ltd
for the loan of yoga equipment.

Special thanks to Rebecca Mercer for six
hand-painted *chakra* mandalas.

*Yoga is about changing the
whole way we think about
ourselves and our world.*

Patanjali, *Yoga Sutras* 1:2

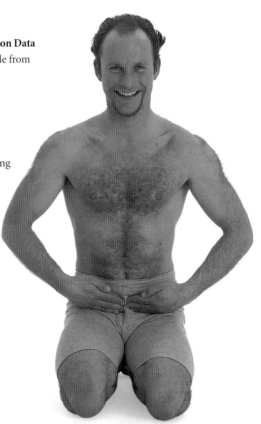

Contents

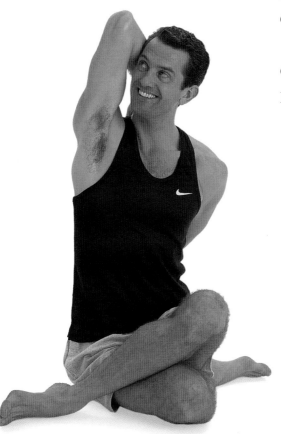

• Precautions

The programmes in this book have been designed to be a safe introduction to yoga. However, neither the publisher nor the author can accept responsibility for any injuries sustained during their performance. If you are pregnant or if you have any doubts about your health, consult a doctor before embarking on any of these techniques.

All yoga techniques work because they focus the mind and stimulate the body.

There are four main classical yoga traditions: hatha yoga, raja yoga, karma yoga and bhakti yoga. As you work through the poses and exercises in this book you will be practising all the major yoga techniques – *pratyahara*, *asana*, *kriya*, *pranayama*, *mudra*, *bandha* and *samyama*. Hatha yoga is thought by most scholars to mean the yoga of balance – *ha* (the sun) and *tha* (the moon). From that derive other notions of balance – left and right; male and female; positive and negative; yin and yang – so it's important that you perform all the poses on both sides and alternate the side you start with.

Yoga is a science of living, and it includes physical movements and postures, skilled and precise breathing techniques, properly structured mental concentration and safe and effective relaxation exercises. Regular practice will help you to become physically fitter, mentally more alert, emotionally calmer and personally more stable and confident about your life.

Yoga works best when it is practised daily, but most people find it hard to set aside a time for yoga every day. There can also be the temptation to make random choices of techniques and to end up performing the same limited range, mostly of postures, without proper regard for their suitability. It's not easy to make genuine progress, and bad habits can easily form, in posture work, in breathing and in the mental techniques.

If you work through the programmes in this book, you will develop a repertoire of postures and techniques that you can build up into a routine that suits your own personal circumstances. If you make the time you spend on yoga special and enjoyable, the benefits you derive from it will increase. As you practise these programmes, remember that yoga is about enjoying the journey just as much as it is about arriving.

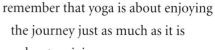

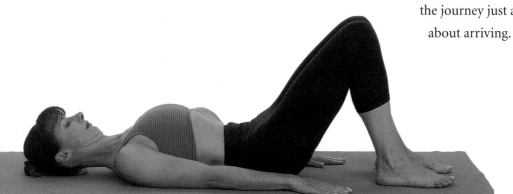

This book aims to provide you with a generous supply of yoga programmes that you can perform at home. The programmes are designed – in pairs – to be a balanced selection of postures, breathing exercises, mental techniques and relaxation (see page 30). If you follow the sequence of programmes you will have a really full and interesting selection of things to do each day, and your expertise and understanding will become deeper and more mature. Each programme is designed to take about 10 minutes. If you can spare 20 minutes, just put the two halves of the pair together – you can leave out the last item in the first, and the first item in the second, and save yourself five minutes.

Yoga is good for everybody, from the earliest years right through to full maturity and old age. It's also infinitely adaptable: we've given you the full versions of all the techniques in the programmes, but we've taken care to show you when and how you should adapt them.

If you have any doubts about whether you should perform something in a programme, consult your doctor. See page 135 for advice about yoga and your health.

There's a complete guide to getting the most from your yoga on pages 32–3, and every programme has a detailed commentary. There's also a full glossary containing the Sanskrit terms. We felt it was important to provide you with the full Sanskrit terms for the techniques, alongside their English equivalents. Quite often, we have given you a selection of English words and phrases, where the Sanskrit is not easy to translate. At the end of the book are some ideas for further study, and suggestions for mixing and matching yoga techniques to make up your own choice of yoga programmes.

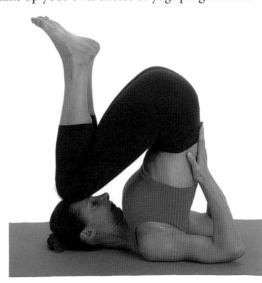

Part 1

Introduction

Before we turn to the programmes themselves, we are going to look at the traditional poses that are used as the starting point for individual postures. There are also a number of limbering exercises, as well as information about hand gestures and aids to performing the programmes.

It's not a good idea to practise yoga techniques when your mind and your body are not ready.

Your mind needs to be ready, so that you can concentrate on what you are doing. We have given you a time to prepare your mind, at the beginning of each programme. The traditional Sanskrit name for this is *pratyahara*, a word that has many English equivalents. We have called this period 'becoming aware'. If you are performing a double programme you don't need to include this period at the beginning of the second part of each programme.

Your body needs to be ready, too. Your joints and muscles need to be warmed and loosened, and if you don't prepare the parts of your body that you are going to use, you will not be supple enough to enjoy the programmes and you could get cramp or injure yourself.

Limbering Exercises

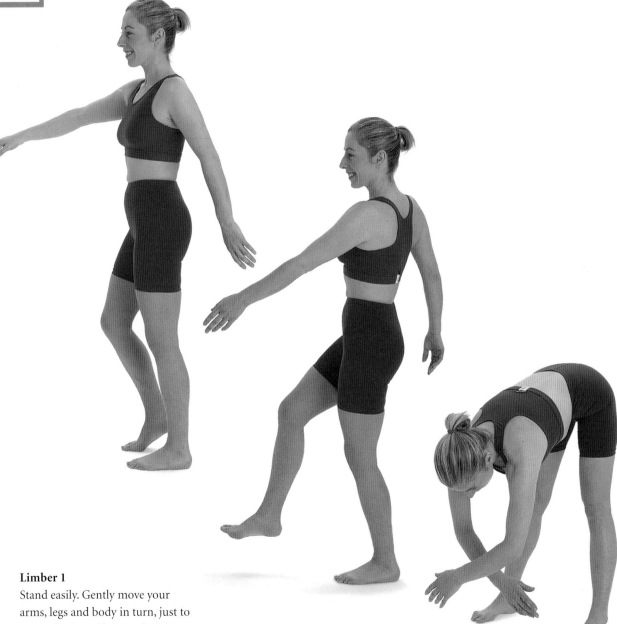

ere are 10 different limbering sequences, each one designed to prepare you for a particular group of postures (*asanas*). Until you get used to performing these sequences, it is suggested that you refer to these pages each time.

After each posture you need to help your body restore its balance and to allow energy to flow through the parts of your body you have just used. A good way to do this is to repeat the limber sequence. Performing a posture an equal number of times on each side will also help. When you come to design your own programmes, you can also group complementary postures together.

Limber 1
Stand easily. Gently move your arms, legs and body in turn, just to warm them, and loosen the joints. Pretend you are a rag doll.

Limber 2

Sit in the centre of your space. Extend your legs out in front of you. Bring your knees up under your chin. Let them fall apart, and gently open them with your arms. Take each foot in turn in your hand. Move it: up and down; out to the side; back towards your shoulder. Return to the sitting position.

Limber 3

Sit easily. Lift your knees to your chest and rock gently from side to side. Lift your left foot and try to straighten your left leg, raising it up into the air. Lower your leg and rest the foot on the floor. Repeat with the other leg. Reverse the order next time. It will help if you slip one hand under each thigh, so that they are free to move separately. Return to the rocking movements before resting.

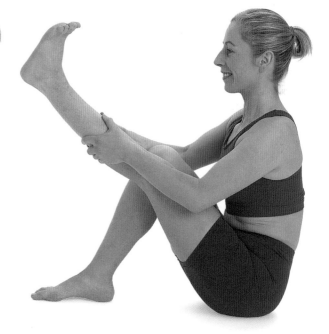

Limber 4

From a tall standing position, the Mountain, inhale. As you exhale, lower your head, bring your shoulders forward, curl your back down, and let your arms hang down so that your hands reach down towards the floor. Breathe quietly and encourage your body to fold right down to its lowest point. This varies, so find your own optimum position. Stay there, breathing quietly – feel your back softening and your legs getting longer.

Begin to uncurl. Make sure that you have seen your shoulders open before you raise your head, inhaling and resuming the Mountain.

Limber 5

Assume the Pole (page 17), taking time to perform it with care and attention. Lift your left leg out to the side, using your hands to minimize the movement of your spine. Do this with your right leg too. Use small movements to ease your legs out to their widest angle. Take your buttocks out behind you, and sit fairly and squarely on your sitting bones. You may feel some of your lazy muscles starting to complain, so don't be too ambitious. Put your hands together in front of you, and 'walk' your hands forwards. Keep your back straight. Your spine will lower and your hips will begin to fold. Go as far forward as your hands will walk. Stay there, breathing gently. This will open your hips, and extend the muscles in your thighs. Return to the Pole and rest. Cuddle your knees to your chest if you like and then go for another walk.

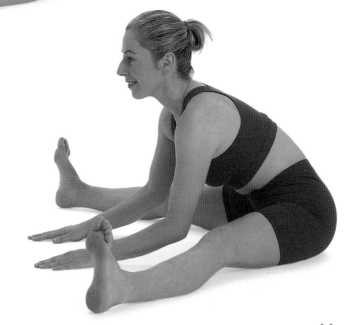

Limber 6

Assume the Pole (page 17) but take your left leg over the right, so the left foot is touching the right knee. Turn and look over your left shoulder, take your left hand behind you for support and place your right hand onto your left thigh for help with the rotation.

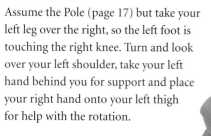

Slowly return to the front, switch legs, and perform the rotation to the right. Repeat this movement several times. Try it quite quickly, but not carelessly. Try it slowly and pause in the turn, breathing quietly. Try exhaling as you turn, so that you turn with a small waist.

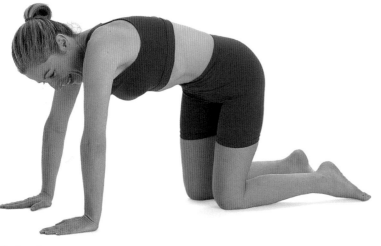

Limber 7

Assume a position on all fours. Make sure that your hands are properly under your shoulders and that your knees are under your hips, or you will not get the support you need. Gently move your spine up and down. See if you can rotate your spine: keep your breathing quiet and move your torso up, then to the right, then down and finally to the left. It doesn't matter if it's not perfect. Rotate in the other direction.

Limber 8

Lie supine in the Corpse (page 18) and bring your knees up to your chest, cuddling them with both arms and rocking gently to and fro and from side to side.

Limber 9

Lie face down on your mat. Put your hands under your shoulders and gently lift up your upper body just a little way.

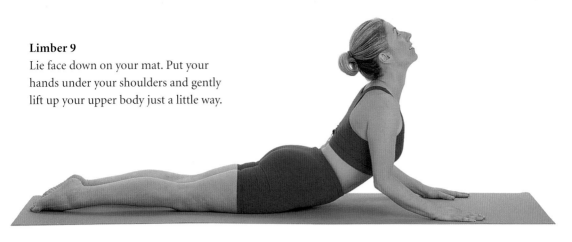

Then let it down again. Put your hands back by your sides and gently lift up your legs just a little way. Let them down again.

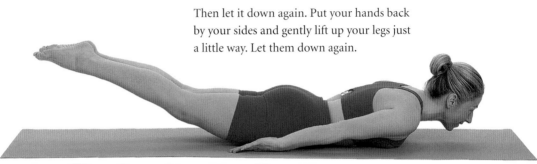

Limber 10

Sit on your mat, with your hands under your knees.

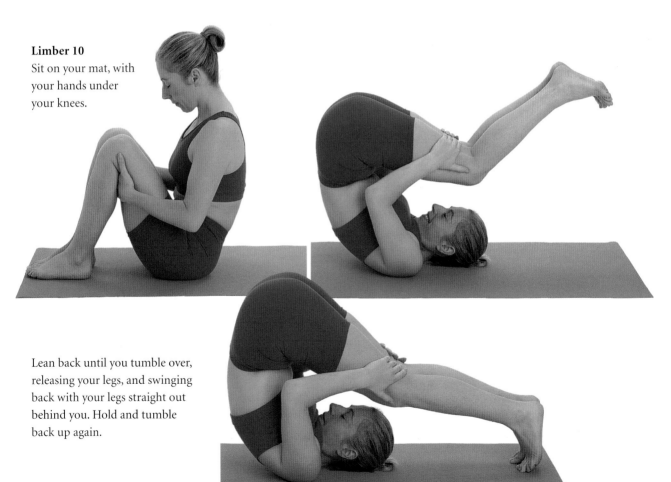

Lean back until you tumble over, releasing your legs, and swinging back with your legs straight out behind you. Hold and tumble back up again.

All the postures (*asanas*) in yoga begin from one of the five classical positions, and most of them return to it. These positions help you to begin the posture with a few moments of calm awareness and to conclude on a note of stillness and control.

In each programme we suggest that you firmly establish the classical position or starting posture before you embark on the *asana*. Use these pages to become familiar with these postures before beginning the programmes that use them. The five postures are:

- **The Mountain,** the true yoga standing position
- **The Rock,** the kneeling position
- **The Pole,** the correct sitting position
- **The Corpse,** total resting on your back
- **The Prone Corpse,** total resting on your front.

The benefits of yoga, physical, mental and spiritual, work best when we are fully aware. These ancient basic positions give us the chance to establish a pose and settle our thoughts, before embarking on a body movement or mental technique.

When we have performed any yoga posture, it's good to return again to the basic position, and collect our thoughts before proceeding to the next event. These attitudes will begin to affect our general lifestyle, teaching us to pause, if only for a moment, before undertaking a task, or making a decision, so that our attention is always focused, and our performance more poised.

This is the real way to pace ourselves, put our energy to the best use, and stay relaxed.

Sthiram sukham asanam.
(Postures should be firm and feel good.)
Patanjali, *Yoga Sutras* 2.46

The Mountain

The Mountain (*tadasana*) is the true yoga standing position. It lengthens the whole body and restores its proper balance. If you have time, when you have completed the pose let your whole body go soft and assume the position all over again.

1 Stand tall.
2 Have your feet nearly touching.
3 Stand equally on your left and right foot.
4 Stand equally on the balls and heels of your feet.
5 Tighten your knees.
6 Stand tall on your legs.

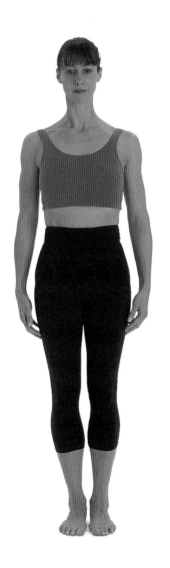

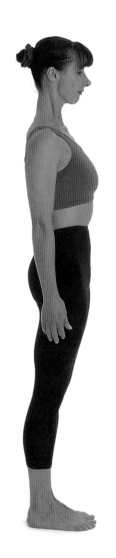

7 Move the front of your pelvis up, and your tailbone down.
8 Lift and widen your midriff.
9 Lift your chest and widen your shoulders.
10 Place your arms beside you, the hands lightly touching the sides of your thighs.

11 Lift your head to the top of your neck.
12 Look straight ahead.
13 Glance down towards the floor.
14 Breathe deeply into the top of your chest.
15 Exhale into your abdomen.
16 Continue breathing gently with your abdomen only.

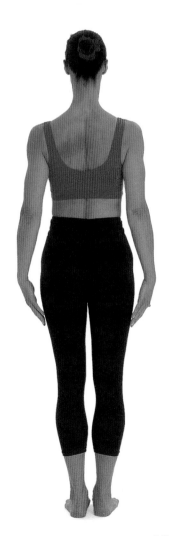

The Rock

The Rock (*vajrasana*) is the basis of the kneeling postures, and it is marvellous for developing a straight back and an open chest.

Stay still in the pose for 12 seconds before resting, enjoying a feeling of inner strength.

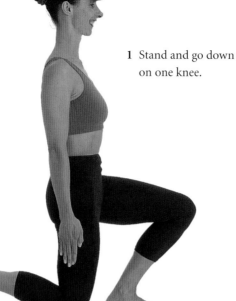

1 Stand and go down on one knee.

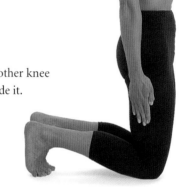

2 Bring the other knee down beside it.
3 Kneel tall.

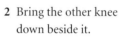

4 Lay your toes down on the floor.

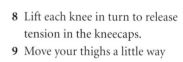

5 Move your torso back horizontally and down vertically, until your buttocks are resting on your heels.
6 If this is a problem, use a kneeling stool.
7 Feel your feet opening out to support your buttocks.

8 Lift each knee in turn to release tension in the kneecaps.
9 Move your thighs a little way apart.
10 Lift the soft parts of your buttocks out behind your heels.
11 Feel your sitting bones.
12 Move your pelvis back to flatten your abdomen.
13 Place your hands flat on the tops of your thighs.
14 Breathe deeply into the top of your chest.
15 Breathe deeply out in your abdomen, leaving your chest up and open.

The Pole

. . . .

The Pole (*dandasana*) is the basis of all the seated *asanas*. Resume the seated position from your limbering and begin to perform the Pole.

If you can, stay still in the pose for 12 seconds. Then rest.

1 Sit tall.
2 Lift out the soft parts of your buttocks to each side, so that you can feel your sitting bones.

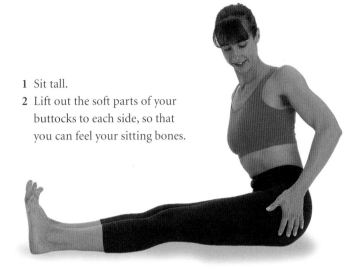

3 Move your legs slightly apart.
4 Lay them really flat.
5 Try to feel the backs of your knees on the floor.
6 Keep your feet vertical.
7 Keep your toes vertical.

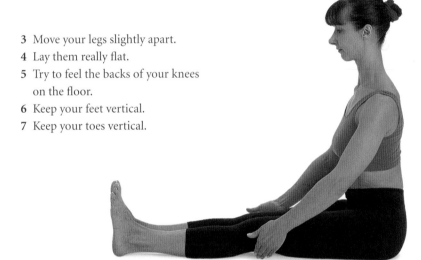

8 Sit really tall.
9 Roll your lower abdomen back over your sitting bones.
10 Lay your hands, palms down and fingers pointing forwards beside your hips, or on your thighs if you can't reach the floor; if you have long arms, sit taller.
11 Look straight ahead.
12 Glance down to your knees.
13 Breathe deeply into your chest.
14 Breathe deeply out in your abdomen, leaving your chest lifted and open.

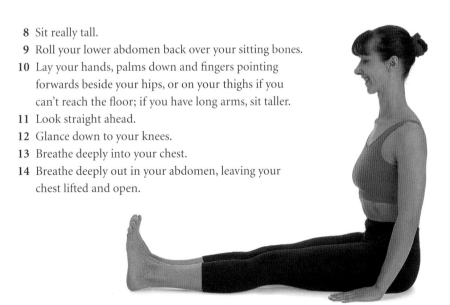

The Corpse

The name the Corpse (*savasana*) refers to the total rest and relaxation that are the main features of the pose.

When the pose is complete, perform several rounds of the Complete Breath (page 35). Rest. If you have time, slip your hands under the small of your back, to help you to return to the Pole, and then assume the Corpse again.

1 Start from the Pole.
2 Reach forward and put your fingertips on your toenails or on your shins or your knees.
3 Lower your head as your back curves forward.

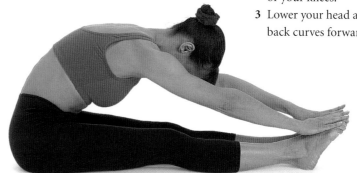

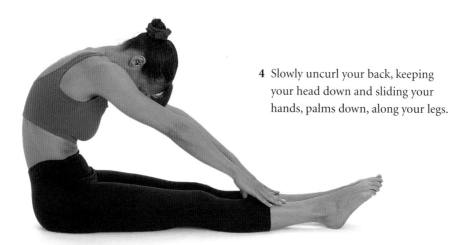

4 Slowly uncurl your back, keeping your head down and sliding your hands, palms down, along your legs.

5 Lie flat on your back.
6 Roll your arms out and turn your palms up.
7 Let your feet turn out and feel your knees become soft.
8 Adjust your pelvis so that the small of your back touches the floor.
9 Adjust your shoulder blades so that the tips of your shoulders touch the floor.
10 Lift your head and lay it down, with your chin tucked in.
11 Breathe deeply into your chest.

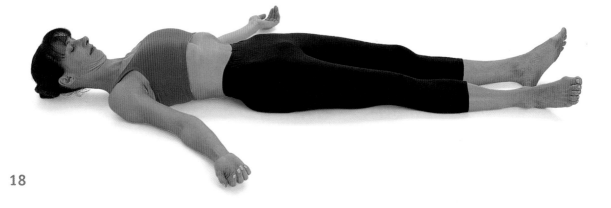

The Prone Corpse

The Prone Corpse (*advasana*) is a precise and powerful way of lying on your front.

Pause in this pose, with your breath held full. As you exhale, let every part of your body go soft again, and turn your head onto the other side. Perform two more rounds of breathing, noting that the Prone Corpse is quite a dynamic technique.

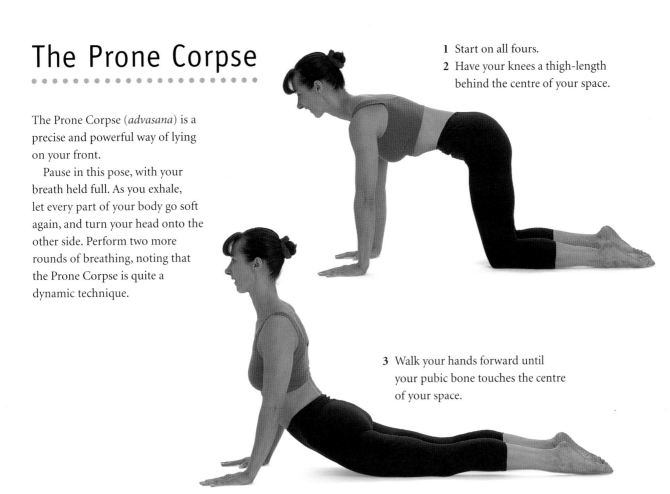

1 Start on all fours.
2 Have your knees a thigh-length behind the centre of your space.

3 Walk your hands forward until your pubic bone touches the centre of your space.

4 Curl down your upper body until you are flat on the floor.
5 Bring your arms up to lie above your head.
6 Let your heels fall out, but keep your toes touching.
7 Turn your head to one side.
8 Breathe quietly.

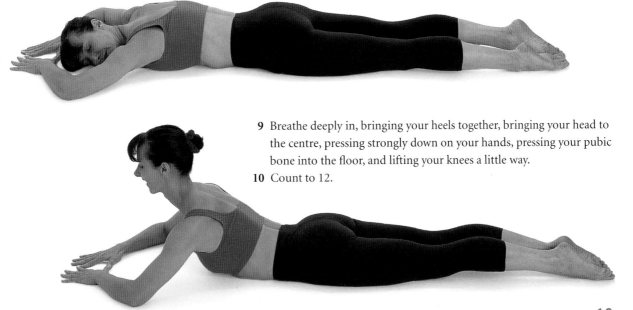

9 Breathe deeply in, bringing your heels together, bringing your head to the centre, pressing strongly down on your hands, pressing your pubic bone into the floor, and lifting your knees a little way.
10 Count to 12.

A meditation posture should be comfortable and balanced. It should keep you upright and alert. The traditional seated postures (*asanas*) are ideal, and on the following pages we explain them for you in detail.

The four postures are:
- **The Easy Pose**
- **The Pose of the Expert**
- **The Half Lotus**
- **The Lotus**.

We strongly recommend you to experiment with blocks. The best sort to use are firm polystyrene blocks, about 5cm (2in) high, 30cm (12in) long and 20cm (10in) wide. A good temporary alternative is a thick telephone directory. Because we tend to sit on chairs, our hips are not very flexible, and sitting in meditation on the mat, without blocks, is just not possible for most of us. So try the postures on these pages with two blocks. If there are no problems, try them with one block – if you are supple you may not need to use blocks at all.

Remember that the postures are not correct, or safe, if your knees are raised off the mat. You should also check that you can sit perfectly upright with your hands in your lap. If you start to tip over backwards, you need more blocks. If two blocks are not enough, you should meditate in the Rock pose, perhaps with a kneeling stool, until you are more flexible. Always sit with the short side of your block under you. Sit on the very front edge.

In all of these meditation postures (*samyama asana*), complete the setting up process with a deep breath into your chest, a deep exhalation into your abdomen and gentle breathing in your abdomen only, keeping your chest lifted and open.

We will explain the hand positions on page 24. Just for now, it's quite acceptable to lay your hands over your knees; remembering to experiment with placing your hands in your lap.

A student of Yoga should sit still,
with his body, neck and head in a straight line.
Bhagavad Gita 6:13

The Easy Pose

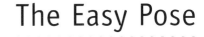

The Easy Pose (*sukhasana*) is suggested for many of the meditations in the programmes that follow. As with all the poses, remember to alternate your legs each time you practise it.

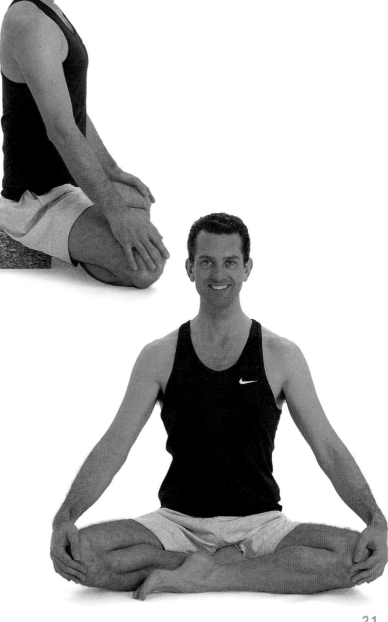

1 Sit with your legs out in front of you.

2 Bring your right foot into your groin, and place its heel against your perineum.

3 Lay your right knee down on the floor, well out to your right side.

4 Bring your left foot to lie alongside the right foot.

5 Lay your left knee down on the floor, to match the angle of your right knee.

6 Sit tall, and perform the breathing sequence (see page 20).

7 To release the pose, gently open the legs, and cuddle your knees for a few moments.

The Pose of the Expert

The Pose of the Expert or the Perfect Pose (*siddhasana*) is reckoned to be the pose for seated techniques for most people.

Make sure that the inner foot is well tucked under, so that the outer foot and leg can lie over it. Release as for the Easy Pose.

Don't worry if it's awkward – these things take time. Return to the Easy Pose and try again next time.

1 Place your right foot against your perineum.
2 Place your left foot in the fold of your right thigh.
3 Sit tall and perform the completing breath.

Remember to alternate your legs.

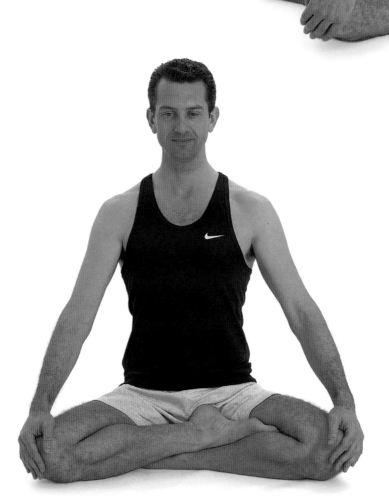

• Precautions

Never struggle into yoga postures, especially these.

22

The Half Lotus

The Half Lotus (*ardha padmasana* or *eka padmasana*) is a demanding posture, and you may need to use blocks as you begin to practise it.

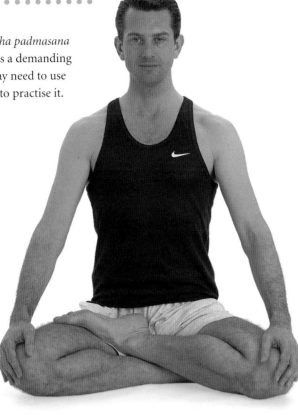

1 Sit with your legs out in front of you.
2 Place your right foot fully against your groin.
3 Lay your right knee down a moderate distance out to your right side.
4 Raise your left knee – you should be able to see your right toes peeping out from under your left thigh.
5 Take your left foot in your right hand (holding it underneath).
6 Lift it up onto your right thigh, letting it turn over so that you can see the sole.
7 Lay the knee down on the floor, at an angle to match your right knee.
8 Complete the pose with breathing as before.
9 Release as before.

Remember to alternate your legs.

The Lotus

You should not try to get into the Lotus (*padmasana*) pose from the Half Lotus.

1 Sit with your legs out in front of you.
2 Bend your right knee, and take your right foot, from underneath, in your left hand.
3 Place it on your left thigh.
4 Collect your left foot, as above.
5 Place it on your right thigh.
6 Sit tall and perform the completing breath.
7 Release as above.

Remember to alternate your legs.

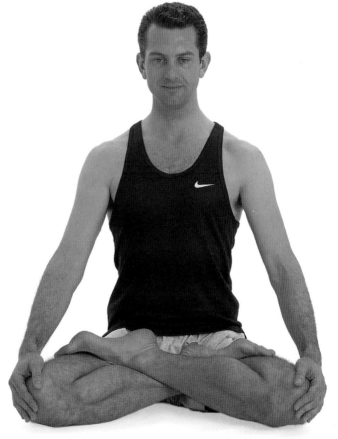

When you are seated in each of the meditation postures you have a selection of hand positions (*hasta mudras*) to choose from. It's important that you choose one of them, rather than let your hands lie idle. If you are using one of your hands, let the other one rest on your knee. Always hold your hands near your body, and if you start to fall backwards, use an extra block.

In these five gestures, an open palm usually means 'being receptive', and a circular shape means 'wholeness'.

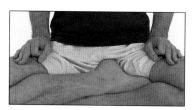

Gesture of Knowledge
(*gyana mudra*)
Have your hands at the tops of your thighs with your fingers pointing towards your knees.

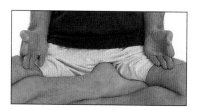

Gesture of Consciousness
(*cin* or *chin mudra*)
As above, but your hands are turned upwards. Feel how much more open your chest is this time. You can also have the pads of your thumb and first finger touching.

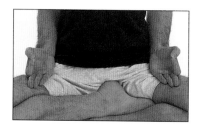

Gesture of Wisdom
(*jnana mudra*)
As above, but have the tips of your first fingers and thumbs touching. The circles you make with your fingers and thumbs represent the wholeness of perfect being.

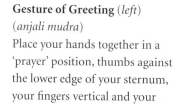

Gesture of Contemplation
(*dhyana mudra*)
Rest your hands in your lap, the right hand resting in the left, your thumb tips just touching.

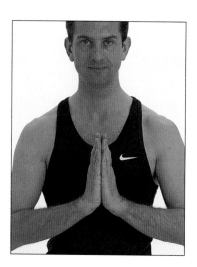

Gesture of Greeting (*left*)
(*anjali mudra*)
Place your hands together in a 'prayer' position, thumbs against the lower edge of your sternum, your fingers vertical and your shoulders down and elbows rested. Press your hands close together. You can also have your hands resting on the crown of your head or between your shoulder blades.

Every now and then in yoga it's nice to get a little help. If you have a medical condition that really limits your ability to perform, turn to pages 135–7 for advice and alternative suggestions. But if you just want a bit of help with some of the techniques, read on.

Blocks

Most of us need one or two blocks when we're learning to sit in meditation. Quite hard blocks are best; see page 20 for details. But aim to reduce the number that you need. Some blocks are not fire resistant; always check before you buy.

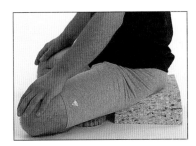

Blankets

If you have a 'bony spine' or a weak or painful neck, it will help to have a blanket under your shoulders in the Shoulder Stand or the Plough. You may also need a blanket under your head for the Corpse pose.

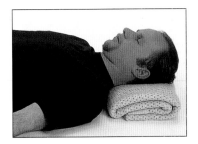

Stools

If you can't kneel, a stool will help. Position it under your legs so that you don't have to bend your knees too far or put pressure on your feet.

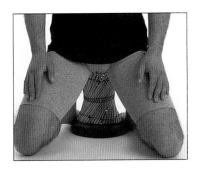

Straps

If you can't reach your feet in the Seated Forward Bend or link your fingers in the Cow's Head, try using a strap to get the benefits of these postures. Regular practice may enable you to do without them; but don't be in a hurry.

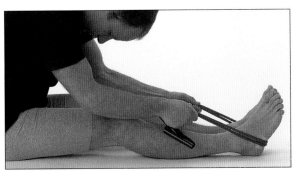

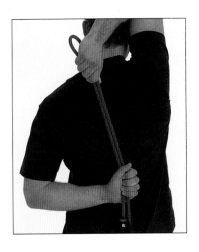

In traditional yoga it's believed that there are seven inner energy centres (*chakras*), which are located in the equivalent of the spine. They generally correspond to the different nerve plexuses. We stimulate these centres when we perform yoga, and we benefit from the energy (*prana*) that they release and that flows along energy channels around the body.

We make sure that these channels are open by performing unblocking techniques, and we help the energy to flow by yogic breathing. We can also direct the energy to special areas by performing locks and twists.

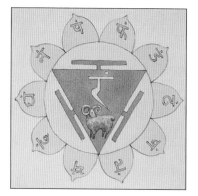

Throat Centre
The throat centre or pure centre (*visuddha chakra*) is located where the neck meets the chest. It is the centre of communication, and its associated colour is blue.

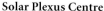

Solar Plexus Centre
The solar plexus centre or city of jewels (*manipura chakra*) is located at the navel. The centre of feeling, its associated colour is yellow.

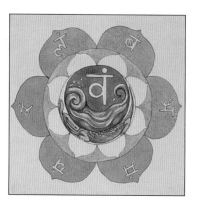

Pelvic Centre or Sacral Centre
The pelvic or sacral centre, the intimate personal centre (*svadisthana chakra*) is located in the sacral area. It is the centre of personal energy, and its associated colour is orange.

The world of *chakras* is enormous, and we can only provide you with a brief account in this book. We hope, however, that it is enough to help you to begin to work with them and to experience their power. In meditations, the *chakras* are usually associated with the colours of the rainbow.

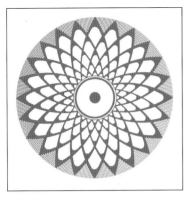

The Crown Energy Centre
The crown energy centre or the thousand-petalled lotus (*sahasrara chakra*) is positioned on or just above the crown of the head. It is the centre of the soul, and its associated colour is violet.

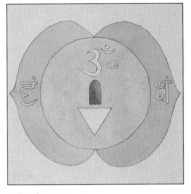

Third Eye Centre
The third eye centre or command centre (*ajna chakra*) is located between the eyebrows. It is the centre of thought, and its associated colour is indigo.

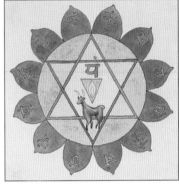

Heart Centre
The heart centre or centre of the unstruck sound (*anahata chakra*) is the centre of love, and its associated colour is green.

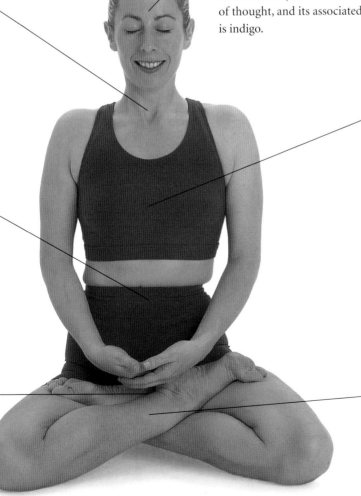

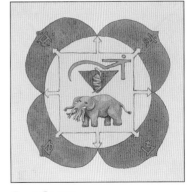

Root Centre
The root or base centre (*mulad-hara chakra*) is located at the base of the spine. It is the foundation of being, and its associated colour is red.

This sequence of movements and positions, known as the Sun Salutation (*surya namaskar*), is rather different from the other techniques in this book. It comes from a time when yoga students wanted something quite dynamic that they could do in the morning and that would take only a few minutes.

It is not a series of postures (*asanas*). It is, rather, more like an extended limbering sequence, so don't treat any of the positions as an *asana*. Move through the sequence smoothly, choosing one of three methods: dynamic, steady or static.

● **Dynamic:** move through the 12 positions, at the rate of one position every two seconds, observing the breathing indicated. Don't linger in the positions – keep moving.

● **Steady:** move through the 12 positions, observing the breathing shown, but not keeping to a strict timing. Linger a little in each position.

● **Static:** move very slowly, staying in the positions as long as is comfortable, and breathing as you need.

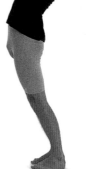

12 Breathe out

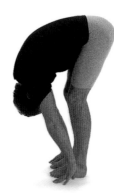

11 Breathe in

10 Breathe out

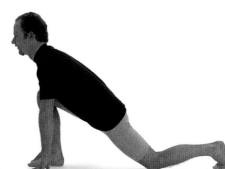

9 Stop breathing

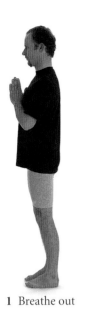

1 Breathe out

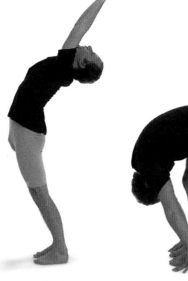

2 Breathe in

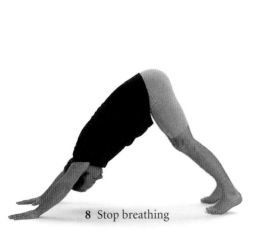

3 Breathe out

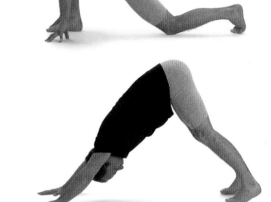

4 Breathe in

5 Stop breathing

Perform it in pairs of rounds, first with the left leg moving backwards and forwards, and then with the right leg moving. If you plan to use it regularly, remember that the sequence provides you with forward and back movements; there are no sitting or supine positions.

You can perform the sequence as a real salutation, especially if you face the sun.

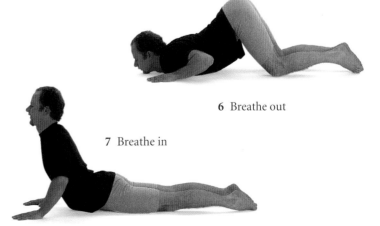

6 Breathe out

7 Breathe in

8 Stop breathing

Part 2

The Programmes

The programmes in this part of the book are arranged so that you can move through them, one by one. The odd-numbered programmes on the left-hand pages are the dynamic ones; the programmes facing them are for breathing, meditation and relaxation. A full yoga experience really requires the performance of a pair of facing programmes.

Try to perform the second part of each programme – those on the right-hand pages – soon after the first part, ideally later the same day or on the next day. If you have time, you can perform the second part of the programme immediately after the first. However, if necessary, it is quite all right to leave it until the next opportunity. It's quite acceptable, too, to miss a day altogether, but remember to pick up your practice with the next programme, so that you continue to move steadily through all the programmes in turn. There is no reason why you cannot repeat a programme, but again, turn to the next programme when you are ready to start moving on again so that you continue to make progress.

Make a note of the techniques from which you derive the greatest benefits, even if they are quite challenging ones. You could include them in your personal selection later.

It is perfectly possible to combine these programmes with attendance at a class. You will get a fresh approach if you do attend a class, for no two teachers have precisely the same repertoire or style, and you may find it useful to get a different angle on some of the techniques. Even so, the programmes in this book are intended to be a complete course on their own.

Programme Title
The orange numbers on left-hand pages indicate active programmes; the violet numbers on right-hand pages indicate programmes for meditation.

Limbering
Preparing the body for yoga practice.

Benefits
The good things that the yoga technique of the programme does for you.

Becoming Aware (pratyahara)
Preparing the mind for yoga practice.

Opening Energy Channels (kriya)
Clearing the way for Inner Energy (prana) to flow.

Breathing (pranayama)
Stimulating the flow of Inner Energy (prana) through breathing.

Meditation (samyama)
Techniques to promote the experience of heightened awareness.

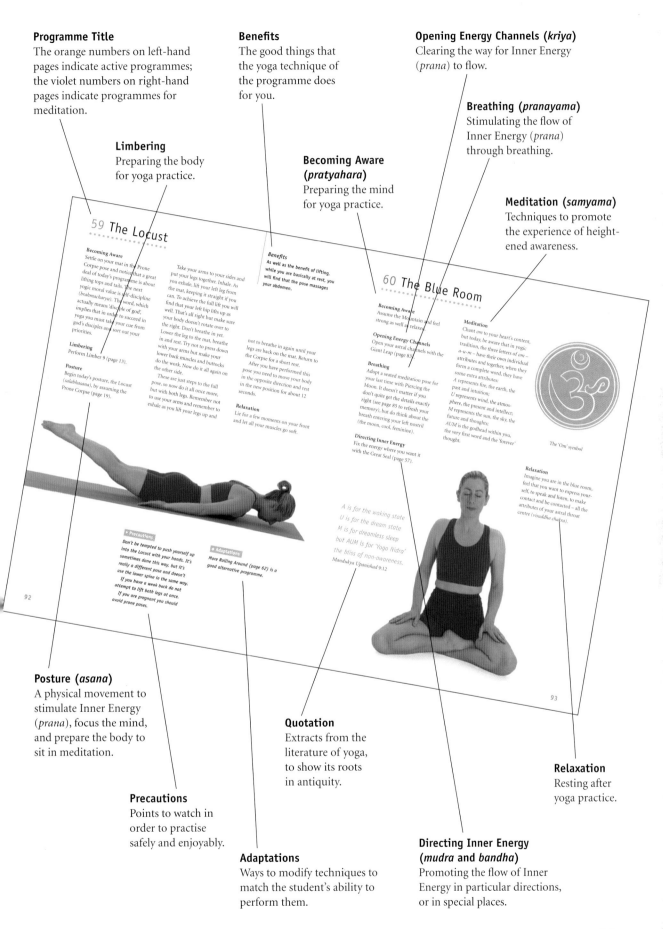

59 The Locust

Becoming Aware
Settle on your mat in the Prone Corpse pose and notice that a great deal of today's programme is about lifting tops and tails. The next yogic moral value is self-discipline (brahmacharya). The word, which actually means 'disciple of god', implies that in order to succeed in yoga you must take your cue from god's disciples and sort out your priorities.

Limbering
Perform Limber 9 (page 13).

Posture
Begin today's posture, the Locust (salabhasana), by assuming the Prone Corpse (page 19).

Take your arms to your sides and put your legs together. Inhale. As you exhale, lift your left leg from the mat, keeping it straight if you can. To achieve the full lift you will find that your left hip lifts up as well. That's all right but make sure your body doesn't rotate over to the right. Don't breathe in yet. Lower the leg to the mat, breathe in and rest. Try not to press down with your arms but make your lower back muscles and buttocks do the work. Now do it all again on the other side.

These are just steps to the full pose, so now do it all once more, but with both legs. Remember not to use your arms and remember to exhale as you lift your legs up and not to breathe in again until your legs are back on the mat. Return to the Corpse for a short rest.

After you have performed this pose you need to move your body in the opposite direction and rest in the new position for about 12 seconds.

Relaxation
Lie for a few moments on your front and let all your muscles go soft.

Benefits
As well as the benefit of lifting, while you are basically at rest, you will find that the pose massages your abdomen.

+ Precautions
Don't be tempted to push yourself up into the Locust with your hands. It's sometimes done this way, but it's really a different pose and doesn't use the lower spine in the same way. If you have a weak back do not attempt to lift both legs at once. If you are pregnant you should avoid prone poses.

+ Adaptations
More Rolling Around (page 62) is a good alternative programme.

92

60 The Blue Room

Becoming Aware
Assume the Mountain and feel strong as well as relaxed.

Opening Energy Channels
Open your astral channels with the Giant Leap (page 83).

Breathing
Adopt a seated meditation pose for your last time with Piercing the Moon. It doesn't matter if you don't quite get the details exactly right (see page 85 to refresh your memory), but do think about the breath entering your left nostril (the moon, cool, feminine).

Directing Inner Energy
Fix the energy where you want it with the Great Seal (page 57).

Meditation
Chant om to your heart's content, but today, be aware that in yogic tradition, the three letters of om – a-u-m – have their own individual attributes and together, when they form a complete word, they have some extra attributes:
A represents fire, the earth, the past and intuition;
U represents wind, the atmosphere, the present and intellect;
M represents the sun, the sky, the future and thoughts;
AUM is the godhead within you, the very first word and the 'forever' thought.

The 'Om' symbol

Relaxation
Imagine you are in the blue room, feel that you want to express yourself, to speak and listen, to make contact and be contacted – all the attributes of your astral throat centre (visuddha chakra).

A is for the woking state
U is for the dream state
M is for dreamless sleep
but AUM is for 'Yoga Nidra'
the bliss of non-awareness.
Mandukya Upanishad 9.12

93

Posture (asana)
A physical movement to stimulate Inner Energy (prana), focus the mind, and prepare the body to sit in meditation.

Precautions
Points to watch in order to practise safely and enjoyably.

Adaptations
Ways to modify techniques to match the student's ability to perform them.

Quotation
Extracts from the literature of yoga, to show its roots in antiquity.

Directing Inner Energy (mudra and bandha)
Promoting the flow of Inner Energy in particular directions, or in special places.

Relaxation
Resting after yoga practice.

The best times for practising are early morning and evening. Some people find that their bodies are stiff in the morning, while others find that their attention wanders in the evening. Experiment to find what suits you best.

- **Always carry out the limbering exercise, even if you find, especially in warm weather, that you don't feel inclined to.** Remember, however, that these sequences are designed especially to prepare those parts of your body that you are going to use in the posture.

- **Do not practise just after a meal.** Try to leave at least an hour after a snack and two hours or more after a main meal. Some people like to have some water handy – and maybe a biscuit – while they are practising.

- **Attend to matters of personal hygiene before practising.** If you can, have a shower, which will help you to feel fresh and supple.

- **Your clothing for practice should be light and loose, but remember to keep warm, especially for the breathing and meditation exercises.** It is best if the room is warm but not stuffy. Ideally, practise in a room where fresh air is circulating but try to avoid a cool draught, especially on you. The room should be sufficiently light for you to see what you are doing – and to read the instructions, of course – but too much bright light could reduce the relaxing effect of the yoga.

- **Make sure there is enough room to practise** so that you do not have to stop to move furniture around. If you have only a narrow space, you can always turn sideways for some of the techniques. You might find it useful, now and then, to use a mirror to see how you are getting on. But do this only occasionally – it's not a good idea to start regularly assessing your progress in this way, and in any case, it's difficult to do most of the techniques and see what you are doing in a mirror at the same time.

- **It is a good idea to have a mat that you use only for yoga,** and this will help you to feel that your practice time is special. Ideally, the mat should be at least 2 metres (6 feet) long and 1 metre (3 feet) wide. You can buy washable, non-slip yoga mats, but any soft washable surface will do to start with. For some techniques you may prefer to work without a mat.

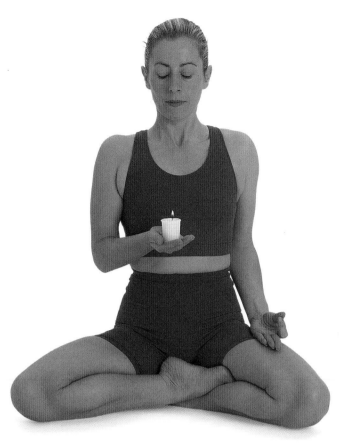

● **Some people like to have a fragrance in the room while they practise and to have a candle burning,** to give a sense of occasion and to help with meditation. Soft music and a clock quietly ticking away the seconds can also help.

● **Regard your practice sessions as opportunities to have quiet, constructive times on your own.** Prepare for them with pleasant anticipation. Perform the techniques with keen attention to detail, but not with anxiety. Be gently objective about your progress, noting your greater and lesser successes and looking forward to your next opportunity to perform those techniques. Think more about style than effort; more about elegance than achievement. Yoga is about travelling, as well as arriving.

● **Most of the posture movements work best with a structured breathing sequence.** Learn the movements first, breathing just as you need. Then add the breathing sequence – and you will really feel the difference!

● **Consider keeping a diary of the programmes you perform,** and perhaps including a note of your success.

● Precautions

Always read the Precautions before beginning the programmes. If you are in any doubt, consult your doctor before embarking on any of the following exercises.

The point of the whole exercise is to become physically fitter, mentally more alert and emotionally calmer. You should begin to have a real zest for life. Take as long as you need to work towards these goals – and enjoy the journey.

1 The Moon

Becoming aware
Feel good about performing this programme and briefly consider what it contains. Settle down and give the techniques your undivided attention.

Benefits
The Moon lengthens and contracts the long muscles at the sides, stimulating the circulation and releasing toxins. But most of all, this posture gently stimulates the whole internal energy system and releases inner energy (*prana*).

Performing this posture regularly will make you feel refreshed and invigorated, but remember that you are only halfway through this first balanced programme – perform the Complete Breath soon.

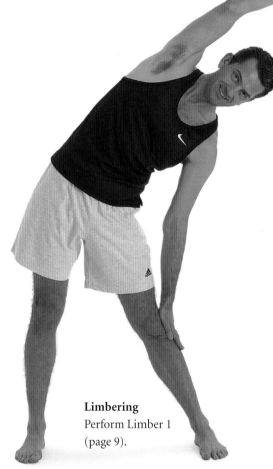

Limbering
Perform Limber 1 (page 9).

Posture
Today's posture, the Moon (*chandrasana*), features standing, so begin by assuming the Mountain (page 15).

Step your feet out about a metre (3 feet) apart, with your toes facing forwards. Inhale and raise your right arm straight out to shoulder height. Exhale and turn your palm up. Inhale and raise the arm until it is alongside your right ear, but not touching it. Exhale and move your arm over your head, moving your head and torso laterally to the left. Go only a little way. Inhale and on the exhalation move your arm a little further. Do not bend your elbow. Breathe quietly and settle into the position for a few seconds, checking that you have moved only laterally and have not rotated any part of yourself to the left.

Continue breathing quietly, and move slowly and elegantly back to the beginning. Do all this again on the other side. Resume the Mountain pose before resting.

Relaxation
Taking care to keep warm, lie down on your back. Breathe deeply and recall the techniques you have performed today.

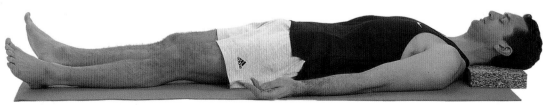

• Precautions
If you find it difficult to balance yourself, find an area of wall big enough to support you.

If moving your arms up is difficult or if you have a back problem, leave your arms beside you in the Moon and bend only a little way to the side.

2 The Complete Breath

Becoming Aware
Sit cross-legged in the centre of your mat (on a cushion if your prefer) or kneel. Briefly recall what you did in the Moon. Settle down quietly and relish the time you are going to spend on your yoga today.

Breathing
Today's programme is about opening the inner energy channels (*kriyas*) and the exercise is Alternate Nostril Breathing (*nadi shodhana*).

Alternate Nostril Breathing
Lower your head slightly and place the first and second fingers of your right hand on the centre of your forehead. Lay your thumb on the side of your right nostril and your third finger on the other side.

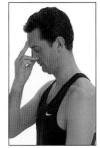

Press gently with your thumb and breathe in slowly and silently through your left nostril. Wait a few moments – notice the stillness. Breathe out in the same way, but through your right nostril. Wait again, then repeat the exercise, but this time start with the right side.

You have now performed one round. If you have time, perform one or two more rounds. At the end, slowly lift your head and sit tall.

Try making the Gesture of Knowledge (page 24) with your hands, so that every bit of you does some yoga.

The Complete Yoga Breath
Adjust your position if you wish. Try letting your knees rest on the mat by slightly altering the positions of your feet and resume the Gesture of Knowledge so that you are in the Easy Pose.

Rest your hands on your abdomen, fingertips just touching. As you inhale, feel your abdomen gently swell and then fall again as you exhale. This little movement will help your lower lungs work efficiently.

Cup your palms around your ribcage, and as you inhale open your ribcage, closing it again as you exhale. This will help the middle part of your lungs to work efficiently.

Benefits
It's always good to settle down and do something easy extraordinarily well, but in this programme you have involved your body in sitting and breathing and your mind in meditation, so you have stimulated yourself in two ways: your blood circulation through the breathing, and your inner energy throughout the programme.

Finally, lay your hands on your upper chest, fingers pointing to your neck, and as you inhale, feel your chest moving up towards your neck, and down again as you exhale. This makes sure that you are using the tops of your lungs properly.

Put all three movements together. Sit really tall, and tighten the muscles of your pelvic floor; this is the Root Lock (*mulabandha*). Inhale in the three parts in turn and exhale through them in reverse. Repeat all this if you have time.

Relaxation
Lie quietly on your back, recalling the techniques you have performed today and listening to your breath.

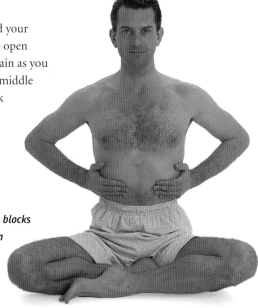

3 Low Forward Bend

Becoming Aware

Briefly send out some good thoughts to your family and friends, and then feel good about devoting the next 10 minutes entirely to yourself. Preview the contents of today's programme, so that your mind and body will then begin to prepare for it.

Limbering

Perform Limber 1 (page 9).

Posture

Begin today's posture, the Low Forward Bend (*prasarita padottanasana*), by assuming the Mountain (page 15).

Step out with your left foot into a really wide stance, your feet facing forwards. Assume a tall Mountain in this new position. Breathe in deeply and begin to bend forwards from your hips, exhaling as you go. Move your bottom right out, keep your back flat and your chest open. If you need support, 'walk' your hands down your legs as you go.

Bend your knees if you wish, but not too much. End up with your hands on the mat between your feet. Pause there, gently inhale, and on the exhalation very gently lower a little further. Drop your head and stay in position, breathing gently, while the pose does all its good work.

To come out of the pose, bend your knees (if necessary) and 'walk' your hands up your legs as you go (if you wish). As you return to standing, inhale deeply and make the Mountain as you come to the top of the pose.

Pause again and decide if you are going to do this again. It's always good to repeat postures if you have time, this time beginning with your right foot. You will find you will be more confident the second time and, usually, more correct, and the movement will, therefore, be more beneficial.

Relaxation

Rest briefly lying on your back and listen to your body. If you are still recovering from the programme, wait a minute or two before getting up and make a mental note to perform more calmly next time.

Benefits

The Low Forward Bend involves bending from the hips, working your hip joint and lengthening your back, which help make you supple in those areas. Being upside down promotes your circulation.

In terms of internal energy (*prana*), moving your tail-bone out will stimulate your root energy centre (*muladhara chakra*), making you feel firm and steady, and opening your chest will improve your thoracic breathing, and stimulate your heart centre (*anahata chakra*), helping you to make good personal relationships or mend those that are faltering.

● Precautions

Do not try this posture if you suffer from back problems. Instead, gently perform a 'rag doll' limbering movement. If you have a heart condition or either of the hernias go only halfway down.

When you assume this pose protect your knees by bending them until you are sure if you need to or not, and use your hands to help you 'walk' up and down your legs.

✳ Adaptations

You can still achieve a useful standing forward bend by gently curling down, pausing while you breathe quietly and curling up again.

Balance: After performing this pose you need to move your body in the opposite direction and rest in the new position for about 12 seconds. You should do this whenever you perform a pose in one direction only (see page 9).

4 Candlelight

Becoming Aware

Walk onto the mat or into your space. For a change, begin with your left foot to promote awareness and balance. Assume the Easy Pose (or kneel) with your hands in the Gesture of Knowledge. Breathe quietly for a few moments, sitting taller as you do so.

Candle Gazing

You will need a candle for this programme, which opens the inner energy channels (*kriyas*). Light the candle and perform Candle Gazing (*tratakam*). Sit tall and breathe gently. Look intently at a small part of the candle flame. Blink if you need to, let your eyes water if they want to, and if they feel tired, gently close them. Feel a cooling and clearing in your sinuses and a clarification in your head. Conclude and remain in pose, breathing gently. Put out the candle.

Breathing

Adopt a sitting position with your legs out in front of you. Begin to breathe slowly and deeply, using your abdomen only. Release your abdominal muscles a little when you breathe in, and draw your abdomen back and up, under your ribcage, when you breathe out. Rest after every couple of breaths. Introduce pauses (*kumbhakas*) at the top and bottom of the breath. These are when the benefits occur – they will gradually become natural. Conclude and rest quietly in the pose.

Waterpipe Lock

In programme 2 (page 35) you performed the Root Lock. Now try the Waterpipe Lock (*jalamdhara bandha*). Assume the Easy Pose.

Sit tall and lift your head to the top of your neck, letting it tip back a little. Begin to turn down, without bending forwards, as if you wanted to look at something on your chest. Feel your chest lifting as you do this and breathe in. Continue breathing by using your new abdomen technique.

To conclude, breathe gently, and lift your head up and a little bit back, straightening it from the chest upwards. The idea of this is to strengthen the effects of *prana* in your upper body.

Meditation

Meditate on the breath, but see if you can begin to notice when your single-minded concentration (*dharana*) changes into effortless contemplation (*dhyana*; in Japanese the word becomes Zen).

Relaxation

Lie quietly, letting the breath move gently to and fro. Relaxation is just 'letting go', physically, mentally and emotionally. Learn to do this in your yoga and you will find that it stays with you through the rest of your day.

• Precautions

If you are pregnant, do not hold your breath for more than a few seconds.

Some people get anxious if they stare at a light – just 'listen' to your eyes and stop if you feel uncertain. If you wear contact lenses, you will know if you should wear them for Candle Gazing.

Be aware of how much breathing you do, and if you start to feel dizzy, rest. Now that you have techniques for deepening you breathing, beware of doing too much.

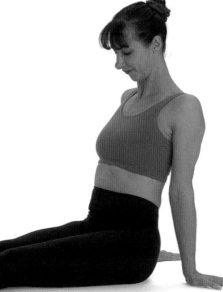

5 Learning How to Kneel

Becoming Aware
Try to become attentive to your programme for today before you actually step onto the mat. Walk to the centre of the mat and feel a real sense of occasion as you arrive at the spot where you always stand and where a lot of your inner energy will be stored.

Limbering
Perform Limber 2 (page 10).

Posture
Assume the Rock (page 16). From the Rock, we will explore the Reclining Rock (*supta vajrasana*). If kneeling is a problem, you can continue from the sitting position you adopted for limbering.

Place your hands, palms down, beside your feet, fingers pointing forwards. Let yourself down, first onto one elbow, and then onto the other. Keep looking forwards, and release your buttock muscles, letting them slip forwards as you arch your back and let your head back and down towards the mat. If you can, touch the mat with the crown of your head, releasing your elbows and placing your hands on your thighs.

If you are able, swing your arms up and back over your head, so that they lie on the mat behind you. Breathe quietly and hold the pose while the *prana* flows and the benefits start working.

Benefits
The posture opens the spine and the chest cavity, which releases *prana* into your upper body. It is superb for sore throats, poor concentration and headaches.

To return to the Rock, place your hands back by your feet, and use your hands and elbows to help you up, lifting your head first. Finally re-establish the Rock. If you have time, perform the Reclining Rock again.

After you have performed this pose you need to move your body in the opposite direction and rest in the new position for about 12 seconds.

Relaxation
Lie flat on your back and breathe quietly.

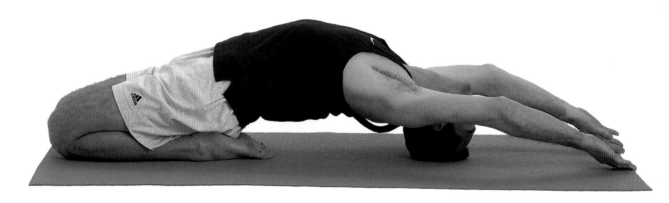

6 Energy Management

Becoming Aware

Assume the Easy Pose with the Gesture of Knowledge. Breathe quietly, sit tall and become aware of your pose and your breathing.

Head-furrow Cleansing

Today we explore Head-furrow Cleansing (*kapala randhra dhauti*), which opens the energy channels (*nadis*) in the head.

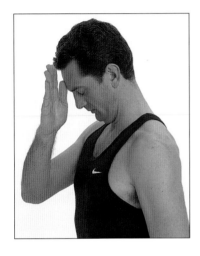

Maintaining the Easy Pose or any seated pose that is comfortable (kneeling if you wish), rest the side of your right thumb on the space between your eyebrows. This is the position of the third eye (*ajna chakra*). Slowly and smoothly move your thumb upwards – you can probably feel a little furrow running up to your hairline. Stop at the hairline and move down again. Do this for a minute or two and then resume the Seated Pose with the Gesture of Knowledge.

• Precautions

Do not perform the Lock that Flies Up if you are pregnant, and go gently with any breathing techniques if you have a hiatus hernia.

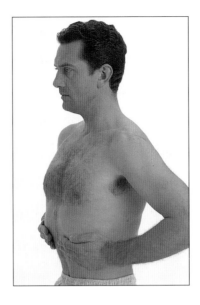

Ribcage Breathing

Assume the Easy Pose again or another sitting position of your choice. Cup your hands around your ribcage and as you inhale, widen your ribcage, pushing your hands apart. As you exhale, gently push your hands together, closing your ribcage again, ready for the next breath. Do not over-breathe, which could cause dizziness.

The Lock that Flies Up

Today we look at the last of the three great inner energy locks (*bandhas*), the Lock that Flies Up (*uddiyana bandha*).

Inhale first and perform the lock as you exhale. You could damage your diaphragm if you perform it with your breath held full. As you exhale, draw your abdomen back towards your spine and upwards, under your ribcage. This is the yogic way to develop the action of inner energy (*prana*) in the centre of your torso.

Benefits

Head-furrow Cleansing can be relaxing because you are performing a yogic caress immediately next to your thinking centre – get a friend to do it for you. The Lock that Flies Up will tone your stomach muscles, and ribcage breathing will improve your ability to use your larynx – it's a traditional breathing exercise for singers.

Meditation

Remain in the Easy Pose with your hands in the Gesture of Knowledge or a similar pose of your choice, sitting as tall as you can. You will forget about your physical body and may find that it has begun to sway, ever so gently. This is good – it's your natural rhythm, which you normally suppress.

Relaxation

Lie down for a couple of minutes and as you inhale, slowly make fists with your fingers. As you exhale, let your fingers go soft again. Nothing difficult about that – and it works magic!

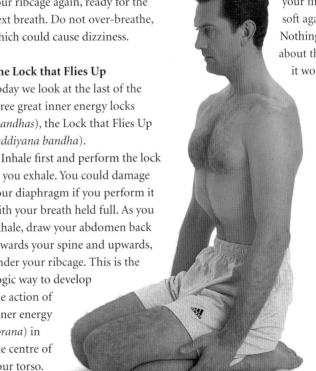

7 The Hero

Becoming Aware
This is your special time, and your mat is your special place. Put yourself first for 10 minutes.

Limbering
Perform Limber 2 (page 10). Make sure that your breathing is evenly balanced. You are performing hatha yoga, which is the yoga of balance and harmony.

Posture
Begin today's posture, the Hero (*virasana*), by assuming the Rock (page 16). Next, slightly separate your knees. Try to do this without disturbing the upright lines of your torso – a hand on the floor between your knees will give you support. Now gently lift your left foot out from under you, and then the right (change the order next time), and see if you can sit on the mat between your feet. Adjust the positions of your knees and feet until you are comfortable. If it is really awkward, try sitting on a block in the same pose or return to the Rock.

To complete the pose, lay your hands, palms down, on the soles of your feet and inhale deeply, sitting really tall. Now you are the Hero.

Bring your hands back in front of your chest, turn them over and link them. Finally, raise your hands way up above your head, inhaling, and with a deep exhalation, turn your head to look up at them. Stay in position, breathing quietly, for about 12 seconds.

To come out of the pose, inhale as you lift your head back, exhale as you bring your hands back down to the soles of your feet, and inhale strongly when they are in place. Bring your hands on your thighs, to rest.

After you have performed this pose you need to move your body in the opposite direction and rest there for about 12 seconds.

This is a busy sequence of movements and breathing, full of heroic gestures. If you have time, do it again and the second performance will be more precise, graceful and satisfying. Feeling firm and happy in a pose is a good guide to the quality of your performance, and if it's correct it will also be safe.

Benefits
The Hero opens the hips, making them more supple and able to cope with the demands we make of them. It also stimulates the root pranic centre (*muladhara chakra*), giving a sense of being firm and steady. The raised arms and linked hands are an excellent way of opening the shoulders and letting breath get to the topmost parts of the lungs.

Relaxation
Lie down for a couple of minutes, briefly recalling what you did today. Breathe quietly, noting if your breathing is balanced. If you find that you are not breathing easily, you may not be entirely fit. Keep a watchful eye on your breathing in the next few dynamic programmes.

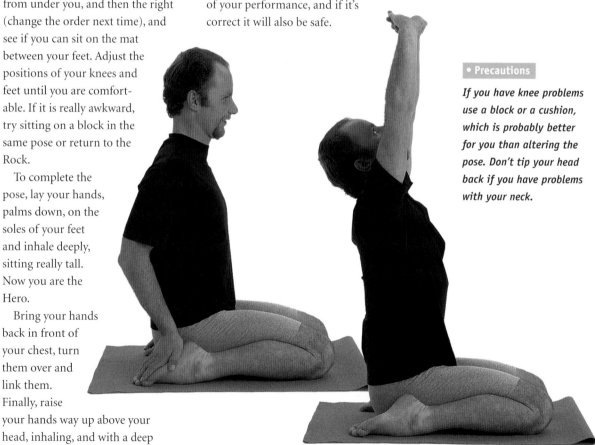

> **• Precautions**
>
> *If you have knee problems use a block or a cushion, which is probably better for you than altering the pose. Don't tip your head back if you have problems with your neck.*

8 The Three Energy Locks

Becoming Aware

Step to the centre of your mat and assume the Easy Pose (page 21). Place your hands flat on the tops of your thighs, inhale deeply, pause and exhale deeply into your abdomen. Remain with your lungs empty (*bahya kumbhaka*) for about 12 seconds if you can, and then resume gentle breathing without disturbing your pose.

Shining Skull

Today's *kriya* is Shining Skull or Bright Thoughts (*kapalabhati*). It will open the energy channels in your mind and help promote clear thinking.

Stay in this pose, inhale and then pretend you are blowing out a small candle. As you puff through your mouth, your abdomen will tuck in (see photograph below). Do this again, but through your nose. Now pretend that it takes five puffs through your nose to blow out the candle and gradually work up to about 12. Inhale between puffs. Remember to keep sitting tall.

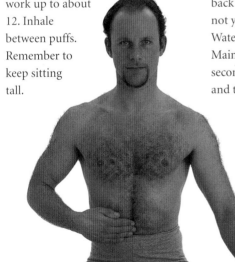

Thoracic Breathing

Resume a good tall Easy pose, your flat hands high up on your thighs. If this is difficult, kneel or sit in a pose you like. Put one hand on your chest (see photograph on right).

As you inhale, feel your chest lifting up towards your chin. Try not to move your abdomen or ribcage. This is thoracic breathing, and it will ensure that you fill your lungs to the very top. As you exhale, let your hand press gently down, to lower your chest. Repeat the exercise two or three times. Make your chest do the lifting, but let your hand help with the lowering.

Directing Inner Energy

Kneel or sit tall. Inhale. With your breath held full (*antar kumbhaka*), tighten your pelvic muscles to make the Root Lock (page 35). Maintain the held breath and lock for 12 seconds (or less). Release the lock and the breath. Breathe gently.

Inhale again. Turn your head back a little and then down – but not your neck – and perform the Waterpipe Lock (page 37). Maintain the lock and breath for 12 seconds. Then release the breath and the lock.

Inhale again. Exhale and as you do so draw your abdomen strongly back and up, to make the Lock that Flies Up (page 39). Pause. Then release the lock and only then gently recommence breathing with an inhalation.

Now perform all three without stopping between (see photograph on right).

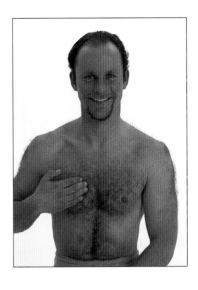

Meditation

Assume the Rock (if you can) and call to mind the three areas you have just energized: your pelvic area, your abdomen and your chest.

Relaxation

Lie quietly and flex your fingers. You will need to return to normal awareness before rejoining your everyday world.

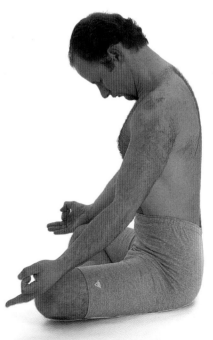

9 Sailing

. . . .

Becoming Aware

The true pleasure of yoga often comes while you are performing, so don't worry if you sometimes take a little longer to get into the mood.

Limbering

Perform Limber 3 (page 10).

Posture

Today's posture is the Boat (*navasana*), a seated pose, so begin by assuming the Pole (page 17).

Lift your knees about halfway to your chin, with a hand under each thigh.

Breathing quietly, tilt your head and torso back so that you are looking up at about 30 degrees. Keep your back straight, breathe quietly, begin to balance on your sitting bones. Complete the pose by lifting your feet to a horizontal position. It's not necessary to stay in the pose too long – just long enough to get the feeling of balance. Then let your feet down and your torso go back to vertical. Rest.

Try again, but this time straighten your legs, so that they make an angle equal to the angle of your torso. You can also release your hand-holds and extend your arms forwards, beside your legs, before coming down again and resting.

You can also stay in the pose for a while, as long as you reserve enough energy to come down elegantly.

After you have performed this pose you need to move your body in the opposite direction and rest in the new position for about 12 seconds.

Benefits

This programme will tone your buttocks in 10 short minutes, but it's also about stimulating the root energy centre and giving you a real feeling of physical and mental steadiness.

Relaxation

Lie on your back and raise your knees. Your feet should be hip-width apart for extra comfort. Notice how this posture moves your spine down onto the floor.

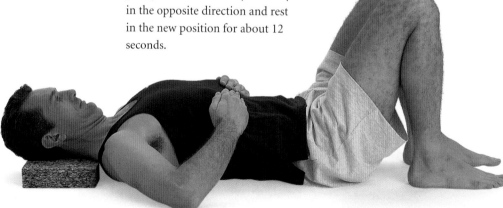

Asanas are the first stage of hatha yoga:

they make the yogi strong, healthy and supple.

Hatha Yoga Pradipika 1:17

10 Dealing with Indigestion

Benefits
This is the classic technique for toning stomach muscles. That's not its traditional purpose, of course, but it does exercise them in a carefully structured way.

Becoming Aware

Assume the Pole (page 17). Give your full attention to your posture, sitting tall as you complete the pose with chest inhalation and abdominal exhalation. Stay in position, holding your breath for 12 seconds if you can.

Breathing

Relax in your seated pose and lean slightly back on your hands, palms down and fingers pointing to the rear. Gently lift and open your chest with a slow, deep inhalation and breathe gently in your abdomen.

Outward signs of progress are a slim and vivacious appearance.

Hathayoga Pradipika
2:19

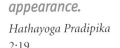

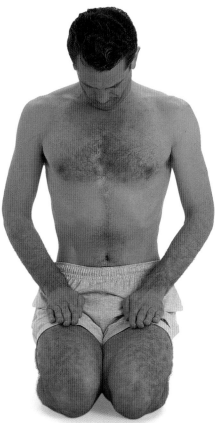

Cleansing with Internal Fire

This *kriya*, Cleansing with Internal Fire (*agnisara antar dhauti*), is about moving the abdominal muscles to promote digestive well-being and to prepare the abdominal pranic channels (*nadis*) for stimulation.

Inhale and look at your navel – it will rise as you breathe in. Exhale and watch it fall. At the end of the next exhalation, pull your abdomen in and release it, with the breath still out. Repeat that, but with two or three pulls and releases, still with the lungs empty, and then inhale.

Always pull first, because that is the main part of the technique. The release is really only to get ready for the next pull. Beware of overdoing it, especially at this early stage.

Meditation

You can release *prana* just by calling to mind an area of your inner (subtle) body. Think about today's exercise and become aware of *prana* moving in your abdomen. The *prana* there is often called *samana prana*. Let the feeling quietly hold your attention.

Relaxation

Lie down, and spend a quiet minute or two wiggling your toes, at first quite vigorously and then more slowly.

• Precautions

Do not attempt this breathing technique if you are pregnant. Some gentle ribcage breathing will do just as well.

43

11 The Tree

. . . .

Benefits
Yogic balances are clever. You can't really do them if you're anxious, but doing them is a splendid way of dealing with anxiety.

Becoming Aware

We're working in the standing position today, so assume the Mountain (page 15). Think briefly about your family and friends and wish them well. Then make a dedication: let this little space in your day be devoted to you and your best interests.

Limbering

Perform Limber 1 (page 9).

Posture

Today's pose, the Tree (*vrksasana*), is a classic standing balance. Balancing is always a challenge, and the best way to achieve it is by not trying too hard. You can't balance if you are anxious about it, and this pose will teach you how to be truly carefree. There are several stages in building the pose, and you can opt to stop anywhere and continue building next time.

Begin with the branches and leaves. From the Mountain, bring your hands up in front of you and join them in the Gesture of Greeting (page 24). Move your hands upwards until they are way above your head and your arms are by your ears (or just behind them if you can), but not pressed against them. Now reverse the whole movement until your arms and hands are back in the Mountain.

Now for the tree trunk. Try several foot positions. For example, rest your left foot on top of your right foot and just feel steady. Try it the other way round. If that's all right, try resting your foot against the side of the opposite knee or on the side of the opposite thigh. If you are supple, try turning your lifted leg over so that it lies, folded, on the front of the other thigh. Try these on the other side too. Decide which foot position you prefer and hold the pose for a short time.

Now for the whole tree. Place your right foot in position (using your hands if you wish). Resume a good standing position – a kind of one-legged Mountain – and raise your hands into their high position. Breathe quietly.

Lower your hands first, then lower your foot. Perform on the other side. If you have time, perform both sides again.

Relaxation

Lie on your back as suggested on page 42 and perform two rounds of the Complete Yoga Breath (page 35). Notice how different it feels when you are lying down.

* Adaptations

If you start to wobble as you perform the Tree, lean against a chairback or the mantelpiece or on a friend's shoulder to steady yourself so that you do not have to break the pose by coming all the way down.

12 Candle Meditation

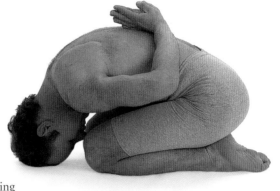

Becoming Aware
Assume the Easy Pose with your hands in the Gesture of Knowledge and be aware and calm.

The Champion's Breath
Today we explore the Champion's Breath (*ujjayi*).

Assume the Rock. Inhale – abdomen, ribcage, chest – then apply the Root Lock and Waterpipe Lock. Pause with the lungs full. Release the Waterpipe Lock, then the Root Lock and exhale – chest, ribcage, abdomen – making the Lock that Flies Up as you go. Pause with your lungs empty, release the lock and continue breathing quietly.

Perform one more round, but this time, as you exhale, lay the second finger of your right hand on your right nostril and exhale only through the left.

Directing Inner Energy
Homage (*yoga mudra*) is a 'body-sign' symbolizing yoga (a rule or discipline). Assume the Rock (page 16) and make the Gesture of Greeting with your hands. Can you put them together like that behind your back in what is called the Reverse Gesture of Greeting? Although it's more correct, it's not compulsory.

Begin to curl your torso down so that the crown of your head gradually comes right down and touches the floor, just in front of your knees. Breathe quietly, and you should be able to settle into the pose for as long as you wish.

The devout feeling you may experience will give you a glimpse of the yoga of devotion (*bhakti yoga*). Curl up again, from the waist, bringing your head up last.

Meditation
Have a candle burning. Return to the Easy Pose and sit really tall and look straight ahead. Concentrate on the candle. Observe the flame closely – its size, shape, colour and movement. Look at the candle-stick, noting everything about it. Look at any shadows thrown by the candle onto the carpet. Try doing this in the dark and see how effective it is.

You will probably find that you tire of the intense concentration (*dharana*) and just become aware (*dhyana*). Instead of 'looking' at the candle, you are just 'seeing' it. Let this happen. Gently return to a state of concentration, blow out the candle and relax for a few moments.

• Precautions

In the Homage, don't stay with your head down for too long if you have a tendency to migraine. If you are pregnant, it will help to open your knees.

Don't overdo the Champion's Breath in case you begin to hyperventilate.

People with breathing problems, including asthma, will find the breathing techniques – with their slow, disciplined movements – a wonderful reassurance. But skill in the techniques can mask asthmatic symptoms, so if you are using a blow-meter, be guided by the reading as well as by how you feel.

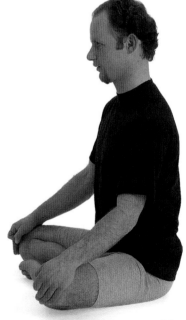

13 The Deepest Standing Forward Bend

Yoga teaches that we have three main ingredients in our characters – wisdom (*sattva*), passion (*rajas*) and lethargy (*tamas*) – but we each have them in different proportions. Which element do you think predominates in your own character? Find out in the next few programmes.

Becoming Aware

Stand in the centre of your space, breathing evenly. Think about this programme and the fact that the aim of yoga is to restore our natural personal harmony.

Limbering

Perform Limber 4 (page 11).

Posture

Today's posture is called Extending the Spine (*uttanasana*). Begin by assuming the Mountain (page 15). Curl down as you did in Limber 4, exhaling. When you have gone down comfortably, slip your forearms around the backs of your knees and place your hands on the backs of your calves. Continue breathing quietly. Now use your exhalations to take just one or two further steps down, bringing your nose near your knees and your hands perhaps on the floor. Don't be too ambitious – remember that everyone is different, in terms of bone structure and muscular freedom. Making the smallest

extension will set all the benefits going. Release the hold and gently uncurl. Repeat the exercise if you have time.

After you have performed this pose you need to move your body in the opposite direction and rest in the new position for about 12 seconds to balance yourself.

Relaxation

It's all right to relax standing up, especially if you don't really want to change your general position. Just curl a little bit forwards so that all your muscles and joints are relaxed.

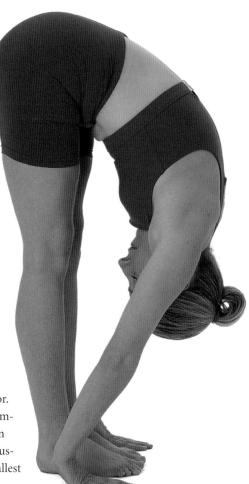

• Precautions

Do not take your head down below your waist if you have problems with blood pressure, a tendency to headaches or either of the hernias. You can perform a similar group of poses from a sitting position.

Listen to your back in these movements and be alert for any sharp lower back pain. If you feel any pain, bend your knees, and use your hands on your thighs for support as you come up.

14 Walking in Space

Becoming Aware

Assume the Rock (page 16), with your palms pressed down on your thighs. Kneel tall and breathe gently in your abdomen. Direct your thoughts to the movement of your navel, slowly out and back. Become aware of the power of this movement to stimulate a meditative mood. This is a popular meditation technique among Buddhists.

Have a tall candle ready. Remain in the Rock and move your tall candle into position for Candle Gazing (page 37).

Breathing

Refresh your skill with the Champion's Breath (*ujjayi*) with the basic technique (page 45). There's more to it than this, of course, but you do need to become familiar with the basics first. Remember that breathing techniques release inner energy and also stimulate and enrich the blood supply to your body, mind and nervous system.

The Space-walker

Can you touch the back of your upper palate with your tongue? Even if you can't, you can still start to learn the Space-walker (*khechari mudra*), which is so called because the tip of your tongue goes on a walk through the space in your mouth.

Adopt the Pose of Expert with your hands in the Gesture of Knowledge. Turn over your hands to form the Gesture of Consciousness (*cin mudra*).

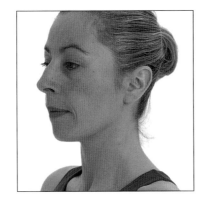

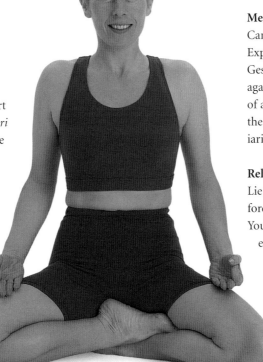

Now 'walk' your tongue to the back of your mouth and try to tuck the tip into the hollow at the top. This is a symbol of collecting or containing the mouth juices, or 'nectar', and preventing them from slipping away. From that idea we get the notion of concentrating inner energy (*prana*) in the mouth and sinuses.

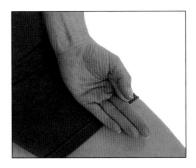

Try to maintain the pose for as long as you can comfortably hold a full breath. Exhale and rest.

Meditation

Can you stay in the Pose of the Expert with your hands in the Gesture of Consciousness? Work again with meditating on the light of a candle, but as always, deepen the experience by using the familiarity to enhance the performance.

Relaxation

Lie down and flex arms. Raise each forearm (from the elbow) in turn. You can inhale as you lift them and exhale as you lower them. As you lie, apparently doing nothing, the benefits of today's programme will be working.

Candle Gazing opens the eyes and cleanses them, so that they work and look better. Space-walking does wonders for sore throats and also helps with breathing allergies. It exercise the mouth muscles and will improve the appearance of your neck. The Pose of the Expert contributes to a feeling of being well seated – a must for good meditations.

15 The Reclining Hero

Becoming Aware

Sit in an easy cross-legged position in the centre of your mat and continue to think about the aspects (*gunas*) of character. *Sattva* means wisdom. Are you sattvic? Yoga teaches that we all have inner resources of wisdom, and when we practise yoga, these are released and we use them. It will become clear in due course if this is your predominant *guna*.

Limbering

Perform Limber 2 (page 10).

Posture

To perform today's posture, the Reclining Hero (*supta virasana*), assume the Rock (page 16). Then assume the Hero (page 40).

Don't perform the hand movements of the Hero now. Instead, kneel tall, your hands flat on your thighs, and perform the usual deep setting-up breath – high into the chest and out by drawing your abdomen in.

Now we are going to lie down in the pose. See if you can lay your hands on your feet and then come down onto your elbows, one side at a time. Lower your back down flat on the mat and your head too, breathing quietly.

Complete the pose by lifting your arms up and back, to rest on the mat behind you. Inhale as you extend your arms back, but don't overdo it. Ease back slightly, so that you are still extended but not strained, and breathe quietly while you feel the muscles from your knees to your chest opening and being refreshed.

To come out of the pose, swing your arms back, to hold your feet. Then slip one leg at a time out from under you and straighten it. Now you are lying on your back and can rest, before deciding if to perform the Reclining Hero again.

Benefits

Opening up your body, as you do in this posture, stimulates the circulation, so that you feel warm and fresh. But your inner energy centres (*chakras*) will be opened too, and the Sweet Centre of the Intimate Self (*svadisthasana chakra*) is especially stimulated. It's in your pelvic area, and is your own special energy centre. Resting afterwards will close it again.

After you have performed this pose you need to move your body in the opposite direction and rest in the new position for about 12 seconds.

Relaxation

It's quite all right to relax in the Reclining Hero and observe how your breathing is restricted to those parts that can move easily – mostly your abdomen. This is a good chance to practise abdominal breathing (see page 37).

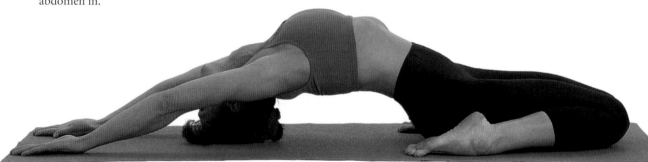

• Precautions

Always listen to your body and learn the difference between the feeling you get when you start using tired or neglected muscles and the pain caused when you hurt yourself. If you have a real stabbing pain while practising, you must stop.

＊ Adaptations

If your knees are a problem, you can sit, rather than kneel, for everything.

16 The Champion's Breath

Becoming Aware

Assume the Rock with your hands in the Gesture of Greeting. The greeting can be for any thing or person you choose, but it may also be for your deep inner self (*atman*), whom you get to meet only when you do your yoga.

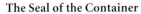

When the breath is still, the mind is still.

Hathayoga Pradipika 2:2

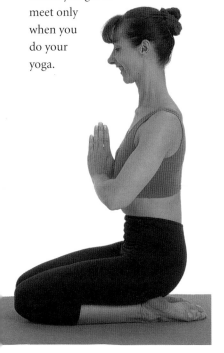

Opening Energy Channels

Perform Head-furrow Cleansing (page 39) to clear the pranic channels in your head and the breathing machinery in your sinuses.

Breathing

Today we will perform the Champion's Breath (*ujjayi*) again, but in the Pose of the Expert with the hands in the Gesture of Consciousness.

The Seal of the Container

Let's stay with the abdomen with the Seal of the Container (*tadagi mudra*) and a welcome change of posture. Slip your legs out to the left side (right side next time) and straighten them, so that you are in the Pole (page 17). Spend a moment or two getting into position.

Bend your torso forwards, exhaling, until you can slip your hands under your thighs or calves. Settle in this position, then inhale strongly and press forwards on the fully held breath. You are compressing your abdomen with the breath held in

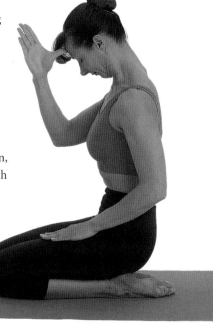

your lower lungs. Only hold for a short time, before exhaling and rising into the Pole again. You can expect to feel powerful in the pose and quite tired for a few moments afterwards.

Meditation

Return to the Pose of the Expert with your hands in the Gesture of Consciousness for another quiet time with the candle. Begin with keen concentration (*dharana*) and just let the rest happen. Meditation starts only when we actually stop thinking. Too much concentration can spoil your meditation.

Relaxation

Lie and twiddle your arms so that the practice confers its physical and subtle blessings.

17 The Lucky Pose

. . . .

Becoming Aware

Sit in the centre of your space. Before we leave wisdom (*sattva*), consider for a moment the yogic notion that it is a kind of perennial tradition – the wisdom of the ancients – and we all carry this with us to some extent. Somewhere, deep down, you have a fund of inner wisdom, and yoga practice releases it. Don't confuse this with knowledge, which we can acquire from books or teachers, or with common sense, which we tend to get from experience.

Limbering

Perform Limber 5 (page 11).

Posture

Return to the Pole (page 17) in order to perform the Lucky Pose (*bhadrasana*). Lift your knees towards you and let them fall apart as they lift. Take a foot in each hand and draw your feet close in to your groin. Try not to lean forwards – in fact, as your feet come close in, sit tall and lift your chest. It will help to exhale as you complete the movement. Notice the way your knees have moved down towards the floor. People differ in this respect, and you should observe where they have got to and gently persuade them to lower a touch further.

Sit tall, breathing quietly. Keep your chest lifted and your abdomen drawn back. Cuddle your knees when you have returned to the Pole to make sure that you are resting the muscles you have just used and that your pelvic energy centre (*svadisthana chakra*) is closed and its energy stored until you need it.

After you have performed this pose you need to move your body in the opposite direction and rest in the new position for about 12 seconds.

Relaxation

Lie down and cuddle your knees, rocking gently from side to side. This will put everything back in place after quite a strenuous programme.

Things that help yoga: enthusiasm, determination, courage and knowledge.

Hathayoga Pradipika 1:16

✱ Adaptations

If your hamstrings just won't let you do the Lucky Pose, sit, leaning back, with your knees lifted and opened. Gently rock your open knees from side to side.

18 Looking at the Void

Becoming Aware

Adopt the Pose of the Expert with your hands in the Gesture of Consciousness. Call to mind your family and friends and send out some good thoughts. Then dedicate this time to yourself.

Opening Energy Channels

Stay in the Pose of the Expert with the Gesture of Consciousness, and perform Shining Skull (page 41). Make the abdomen movements as small as you can, without losing the rhythm or the style. Try to make little punchy tugs of the muscles around your navel with exhalations, with little automatic inhalations between them. If the movements are small, you can make them quicker – aim for about two a second.

Breathing

In today's Champion's Breath (*ujjayi*) keep your eyes closed and complete the technique without thinking about it.

Directing Inner Energy

We are going to practise the Seal of the Void or Looking at the Void (*boochari mudra*). Sit tall and breathe gently throughout. Put your right thumbnail on the tip of your nose and lift your little finger so you can focus on it. Spend a few moments getting this right. Blink when you need to, but you will probably find that as you get used to it, you won't need to.

Put your hand back on your thigh, in the Gesture of Consciousness, and continue looking at the space where your little finger was. Close your eyes when they get tired or your focus changes to

normal and perform the exercise again. The *prana* behind your eyes is stimulated and your subtle awareness is heightened. It actually works best if you sit facing a blank wall.

Meditation

Sit tall in the Pose of the Expert and concentrate on your candle. Let contemplation gradually affect you and maybe you will feel the deep joy that is the sign of yogic bliss (*samadhi*). Most of the yoga that we do is meant to 'put us back together', but there is a further, more important stage when we begin to be less aware of 'us' and start to 'float away on the universal ocean'. Remember that your meditation is not over until you have passed back through the three stages – yogic bliss, contemplation and concentration.

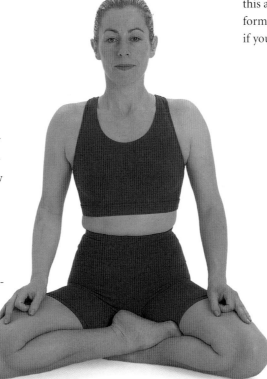

Relaxation

Lie on your back and lift your left knee (right knee first next time) to your chest, breathing gently. Put it down again. Repeat with the right knee. Finally, raise both knees. Do this again if you wish: you can perform this up to three or four times if you are not in a hurry.

• Precautions

Looking at the Void can be awkward if you normally wear glasses or contact lenses. Try gazing steadily at something in your field of vision. Don't stare too hard if you have a tendency to headaches or have things on your mind.

19 Rolling Around

Becoming Aware

Spend a moment becoming attuned to what you are going to do, then walk slowly but purposefully to your space and sit in the centre. Choose a way of sitting down that you can do gracefully. If you really enjoy the postures, you may be predominantly a rajasic person – full of 'get up and go' – or maybe your *rajas* comes to the surface only now and then.

Benefits

This programme is perfect for bad backs, but take all the movements gently – encouraging rather than forcing your body to move.

The rotation massages your internal organs and tones the muscles around your waist. It imitates the spinning motion traditionally associated with the inner energy centres (*chakras*), and so stimulates the whole length of your spine – in one quite leisurely movement.

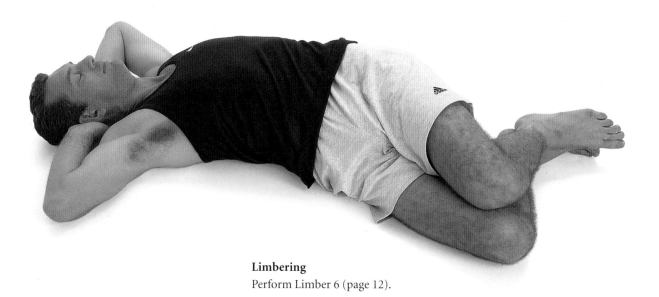

Limbering

Perform Limber 6 (page 12).

Posture

At last we are going to lie down to perform Turning the Abdomen Over (*jatara parivartanasana*). Do it the traditional yoga way by assuming the Corpse (page 18).

Lift your knees so that your feet are flat on the floor and put your hands under your neck. Inhale. As you exhale, let your knees drop over to the right, taking your torso over in a full body rotation. Try to keep your knees together. Let your left shoulder come up a little if necessary.

Stay in the pose, letting it work its benefits right down your spine.

Expect the return movement to be quite challenging. When your knees are back up, look down and check that your body is straight, before performing the posture on the other side. See how the limber prepared your body for this and notice how you use the weight of your own body to achieve the pose.

Relaxation

Your body needs to 'unwind' (literally), so lie and cuddle your knees, feeling your vertebrae settling down again, but in their new, healthier and more supple positions.

20 The Third Eye

Becoming Aware

Assume the Pole (page 17), but lean gently back on your hands. Look down and watch as you breathe deeply into your chest and out from your abdomen. Then restrict your breathing to small movements of your navel. Remain like this as you 'detach yourself' from everything else but your yoga for today.

Breathing

Stay in the Pole and perform Cleansing with Internal Fire (page 43). You will quickly recall the details as you perform the first round. Perform a second round, paying more attention to the quality of the techniques involved – make the exhalation deep, and the pulls and releases of your abdomen quite 'punchy', and try for a rhythm of one a second. Remember to keep your lungs empty while you are performing the pulses. Aim for about 12 pulses, but if you cannot fully control the inhalation at the end, you should reduce the pulses to six. On this occasion, look for the last time for a while at the Champion's Breath (page 45).

The Seal of Shiva

Today we will direct our Inner Energy with the Seal of Shiva (*sambhavi mudra*). Assume the Pose of the Expert with your hands in the Gesture of Consciousness. Sit tall and look straight ahead. Breathe gently and keep your head still. Focus on a point level with your eyes. Now lift your focus by about 15cm (6in) and pause. Do this again and again, until you are looking up under your eyebrows, and at a point as near as you can to your 'third eye' (the point between your eyebrows where Shiva is thought to reside). You may not need to perform all those steps but just do it straight away. Your eyes will soon tire. When you are ready,

either close them and let the focus change by itself or lower your focus back through the steps you took on the way up.

In addition to thoroughly opening your eyes, this exercise will also bring on a strong meditative mood.

Meditation

This is the last meditation with a candle for a while. You may find that you do not need to concentrate and can go straight to contemplation. Contemplation (*dhyana*), the passive awareness of the candle, may just begin as you feel yourself coming under the spell of the candle. Go with it and feel good somewhere deep down in your inner self, where you can't really make out what's happening – do you really need to know? If you get too curious, you will break the spell. Be careful to take the three steps out of your meditation – yogic bliss, contemplation and concentration.

Relaxation

Adopt the Corpse and flex your legs languidly and lazily.

Dhyana is when your thoughts about an object become continuous and effortless.
Patanjali, *Yoga Sutras* 3.2

21 The First Warrior

Becoming Aware
Assume the Mountain with your hands in the Gesture of Greeting (page 24). Pause in this tall, alert pose and think again about *rajas*, which can mean 'passion' in the sense of enthusiasm or in the sense of energy, or can describe a person whose decisions are ruled by the heart rather than the head. If you are exhilarated by postures and breathing, you may be predominately rajasic.

Limbering
Perform Limber 1 (page 9).

Posture
Today's posture, the Warrior (*virabadhrasana*), is named after a great hero, Virabhadra. Begin by assuming the Mountain (page 15). With left foot first (right foot first next time), step out to a wide stride – you will know if this is the right distance only when you perform the pose. Turn your left toes out, by rotating on your left heel. Turn your right heel out by rotating on your right toes. This sounds complicated, but it's to make sure that your left heel is in line with the arch of your right foot and you can balance. Check that you are standing tall and breathing quietly – some people forget to breathe in the more complicated postures. Also check that your torso hasn't turned to the left. You should start to feel that you are extending your hamstrings.

Bend your left knee. If your legs are the correct distance apart, your left thigh will be horizontal and your left shin vertical. If not, remember to adjust the distance when you perform on the other side. Raise your arms to shoulder height. Inhale. As you exhale, turn your head fully to the left and look along your arm. Inhale. Turn your head to the front, exhale and then turn to look along your other arm. Return to quiet breathing. Lower your arms, straighten your left leg, turn your right foot to the front, then to the left and rest with your legs still wide.

If you are tired, sit down and cuddle your knees. But try to stand again after a few moments, because you should really perform the other side.

Benefits
This is the first posture to address the question of stamina, which, with suppleness, is a central feature of yoga. If you breathe properly in the pose, you will send energy to your muscles just when they need it.

To perform on the right side, adjust your legs if necessary. Do not have your bent knee out beyond the position of your foot – you could damage yourself – and to avoid this, you may have to go wider than you think you can. If your knee is hardly bent, you will not get the exercise or the benefits – strong supple thighs and an increase in general stamina – you are seeking.

Relaxation
Why not let your body choose? What would you really like to do? Whatever it is, do it with skill.

• Precautions
If you have weak or damaged knees do not attempt this posture. The Moon (page 34) is an excellent alternative.

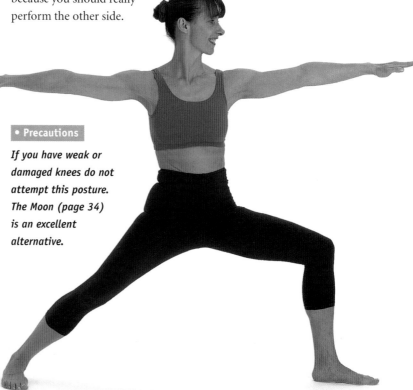

22 Inner Energy

Becoming Aware
Assume the Rock (page 16), with your hands flat on the tops of your thighs. Exhale and stay with your lungs empty for 12 seconds, if you can, with your attention firmly fixed on how the pose feels.

Breathing
Remain in the Rock to perform Alternate Nostril Breathing (page 35).

The Seal of the Six Openings
In this pose, the Seal of the Six Openings (*san mukhi mudra*), you will begin to hear your inner sounds, your body working and subtle sounds connected with your pranic system.

Assume the Pose of the Expert with your hands in the Gesture of Consciousness (see page 51). Put your thumbs gently into your ears, close your eyes and lay your first fingers on your eyelids. Fit your middle fingers into your nostrils and your fourth fingers on your closed lips (see photograph below). Release your nostrils just briefly when you really need to breathe.

Stay in the posture for a few moments and then release your fingers in the reverse order, beginning with your lips.

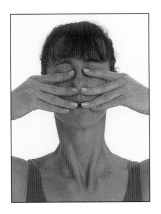

Put your hands back into the Gesture of Consciousness and rest.

When you release this position, your real-life senses will be wonderfully enhanced. Perform it again and enjoy it.

Meditation
Stay in the Pose of the Expert with your hands in the Gesture of Consciousness. Have a candle if you wish; it will help you to focus your mind and keep you company as you meditate. Close your eyes, sit tall and breathe softly in your abdomen.

Imagine that you can see into your subtle body. See a bright energy channel starting at your tailbone and reaching right up to your forehead. It may look pure white. We call this the Gracious Channel of Inner Energy (*sushumna nadi*).

Now see along its length, starting from the base, centres of pranic

If all our thinking about *prana* and *chakras* is new to you and a bit disconcerting, don't worry because it will do just as well to think about your breathing stimulating your circulation and toning your nervous system, which also works through the spine and nerve plexuses in much the same places.

energy: *muladhara chakra* at the base of your spine, *svadisthana dhakra* at the level of your pelvic area, *manipura chakra* at the level of your navel, *anahata chakra* at the level of your heart, *visuddha chakra* at the level of your neck, *ajna chakra* at the level of your forehead and *sahasrara chakra*, at the crown of your head. Observing the *chakras* like this will stimulate them, so you must now go down through them again, starting at the top, to close them.

Relaxation
Stay as you are or assume the Corpse position. Put your palms over your eyes and feel the warmth of your hands and of your eyes, too. This is partly your physical energy, but also a lot of *prana* from today's programme.

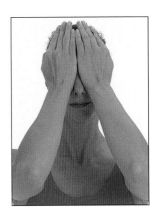

23 The Second Warrior

Becoming Aware

Sit in the centre of your mat and collect your thoughts. You will be starting to be comfortable with the idea that this is your special time and, as you work through the programmes, have a real feeling of calmness. The third *guna* is lethargy (*tamas*). We tend to think of this as a weakness, but how are you going to relax if you do not have any of this characteristic in your personality? When we do our yoga practice, the characteristics fall into the correct balance for us and we regain our natural harmony.

Limbering

Perform Limber 1 (page 9).

Posture

Today's posture is a different version of the Warrior (*virabhadrasana*). Assume the Mountain (page 15), and move to a wide-stride posture – don't forget the completing breath – and have your feet at least as wide as you did for the First Warrior (page 54). Turn your right toes out by pivoting on your right heel, and your left heel out by pivoting on your left toes. Do not rotate your torso. If you did, turn it back fully to the front. You should feel a healthy extension happening in your hamstrings.

Bring your hands into the Gesture of Greeting. Inhale. Turn your torso fully to the right, glancing down to check that your right foot is fully turned out. Inhale. As you exhale, bend your right knee, checking that your thigh is horizontal and your shin is vertical. If they are not, remember to correct it when you perform on the other side. If your knees won't let you do this, perform the Tree (page 44) instead.

Maintaining the position and looking straight ahead, move your hands upwards, until they are straight up above your head with, if you can, your arms just behind your ears but not touching them.

It will feel right to inhale as you make this arm movement. As you exhale, tip your head back to look at your hands. Pause in the position for just a few moments. Inhale as you tip your head forwards again. Exhale as you bring your hands back to the Gesture of Greeting. Inhale as you straighten your leg. Exhale as you turn to the front, and breathe quietly as you resume a wide-stride Mountain posture, before repeating on the other side.

Relaxation

After the strenuous demands of today's programme you will get the most relief if you assume the Corpse and cuddle your knees into your chest, rocking a little from side to side and to your chest and back. This will release your back and rest your knees.

• Precautions

If you find this posture too strenuous, do the Tree instead. You must never over-stretch any part of your body or you will do yourself harm. You will certainly risk damaging your knees if you take them beyond the line of your feet when you bend them.

24 The Colours of Inner Energy

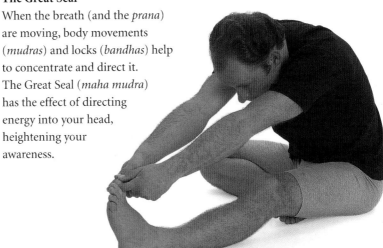

Becoming Aware

You will need a candle for Candle Gazing. If you have strong toes, assume the Rock with your toes tucked under you. You only have to stay in position for a while as you focus on today's programme.

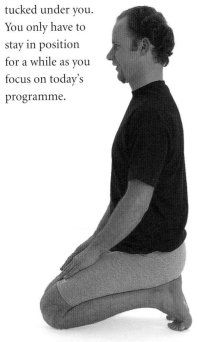

Opening Energy Channels

Slip your toes out and assume the Rock. Focus on the candle (page 37) and see if you get an image of the flame on your retina so that you still seem to see the candle even when your eyes are closed.

Breathing

As we explore the more complex breathing techniques you will find a quietly ticking clock useful. In the Cooling Breath there are four breathing movements. Inhale through your extended curled tongue; hold the breath full; exhale through your nose; wait with your lungs empty. If we call these 'in', 'hold', 'out' and 'wait' – try to time them as follows: in for 4 seconds, hold for 8 seconds, out for 8 seconds and wait for 4 seconds. Rest and prepare for the next round.

The Great Seal

When the breath (and the *prana*) are moving, body movements (*mudras*) and locks (*bandhas*) help to concentrate and direct it. The Great Seal (*maha mudra*) has the effect of directing energy into your head, heightening your awareness.

Assume the Pole (page 17) but fold your lower right leg so that the foot is well into your groin, the heel pressed onto your pubic bone. Inhale. On the exhalation reach your arms out towards your left foot, and grasp your left big toe with the first fingers of both hands, the left hand on top.

If that was an effort, stay in the position until the muscles you are using have softened.

Inhale again, and with the breath held full, flex your foot forwards and look quite hard at your toenails, lowering your head and looking out from under your eyebrows.

Stay for 6 seconds if you can, and then release the breath, the fingers and the pose, returning to a good Pole position, before performing on the other side.

Meditation

Assume the Pose of the Expert with the Gesture of Consciousness. Become aware again of the bright channel of energy (*sushumna nadi*) running up the line of your spine and call to mind again the pranic centres (*chakras*) along the way.

A popular way of doing this is to 'see' colours glowing at the centres as you awaken them: red at the energy centre at the base of your spine (*muladhara chakra*), orange in your pelvis (*svadisthasana chakra*), yellow at your navel or solar plexus (*manipura chakra*), green at your heart centre (*anahata chakra*), blue at your throat centre (*visuddha chakra*), indigo at your brow centre (*ajna chakra*) and violet at your crown centre (*sahasrara chakra*). Hold the colours in your mind's eye, for about two breaths each, as you work up *sushumna*, but remember to work down again, and see the colours fading as you close the *chakras* down. Doing this is yogically the perfect way to flood yourself with pranic, or nervous energy every day!

Relaxation

Lie in the Corpse, breathing quietly, and 'palm' your eyes. Gently stroke your eyelids. Alternatively, you can do a little Head-furrow Cleansing (page 39).

25 The Cat

Becoming Aware

Assume the Mountain (page 15). Bow your head slightly, to make a gesture of greeting. Being able to be calm and collected when all around you is chaotic is good for you and helpful to everybody else. But do expect now and then to feel relaxed – even drowsy – when you would rather not.

Limbering

Perform Limber 7 (page 12).

Posture

To begin today's posture, the Cat (*marjariasana*), assume the Rock (page 16). Move carefully forwards onto all fours. Make the movement more attentive than you did in limbering, retaining control and trying to arrive at the correct places for your hands and feet without needing to adjust them.

Assume what we can call the neutral position – looking down to the floor with your back naturally flat, and not flexed up or down. Inhale gently. As you exhale slowly and deeply, begin to arch your back, from the tail-bone upwards. As the arching movement reaches your neck, lower your head and look under yourself, right through your legs. Pause in this position.

✱ Adaptations

Sit in the Pole and lean back. Try leaning back on your elbows, and arching over them towards the floor. Widening your elbow positions may give you space to touch the floor with your head.

As you begin to inhale, slowly and deeply, begin to move the lowest part of your spine down. Gradually lower all your spine down, until you reach your chest. Lift your head, and look well up. Pause in this position. Now you are ready to start again with the exhalation.

Always begin the movements at the base of your spine and 'ripple' up to your head. It's important that

you move your vertebrae, bone by bone, in this upward direction, waiting until the 'ripple' has reached the top before moving your head. Perform this exercise about 10 times.

Relaxation

Lie face down. This can be restful, and we will explore it more fully on page 82.

Benefits

The Cat is the programme for bad backs because you can make it anything you want, especially a slow movement of the vertebrae combined with breathing. Don't spend too long in one position. Stop when your wrists begin to feel tired.

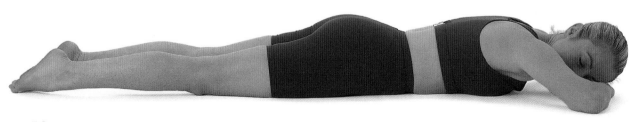

26 The Big Poker

Becoming Aware

Assume the Pose of the Expert but today place your hands with the tips of your thumbs and first fingers touching. This is the Gesture of Wisdom (*jnana mudra*).

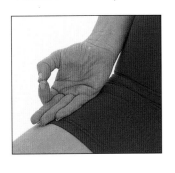

Opening Energy Channels

Maintain your position and perform Head-furrow Cleansing (page 39).

Breathing

Still in the Pose of the Expert with your hands in the Gesture of Wisdom, perform the Cooling Breath (page 57). Today, try a pattern of in 6, hold 12, out 12, wait 6 – that is, 6-12-12-6. If the new count is too much, leave it until later, but don't forget it.

Directing Inner Energy

Explore the Easy Pose with the minimum of blocks and settle for a height that you can just manage.

Today's posture is the Big Poker (*maha bedha*). Seated in a tall Easy Pose, put your palms on the floor at each side and push yourself a tiny bit up from the blocks.

Suddenly, let go and bounce down again. The blocks will push up under you and you will feel a powerful movement upwards, inside you.

This is the knock-on effect of the bounce on your muscles, but also an upward rush of energy (*prana*).

You can perform one or two more rounds, but no more. Try to pause in the lifted position and exhale as you drop down.

Meditation

Choose a seated position that you like and sit up tall, with a deep inhalation. Breathe calmly, preparing yourself for meditation, and visualize the central energy column in your spine (*sushumna*). See energy moving dynamically upwards and slowly settling down again. You can even see the *prana* taking on the colours of the *chakras* it passes (see page 57), but use as little detail as possible, training yourself to fall naturally into contemplation (*dhyana*), the effortless passive awareness of *prana*.

Relaxation

Today we begin to learn about deep yogic rest (*nidra*). This form of relaxation involves being totally engrossed in something pleasant but without consciously thinking about it – just reacting naturally. Assume the Corpse (page 18) and really settle down. Imagine you are walking along a country lane in spring. See spring flowers along the hedgerows but don't feel any need to form any thoughts about them. Hear birds singing but don't form thoughts – just hear them. Smell fresh rain as the sun warms it on the grass in the meadows – breathe it in. Taste the cool breeze on your lips. Feel the breeze lifting your hair. Imagine all these sensations together. Take a moment or two to 'wake up' before concluding your programme.

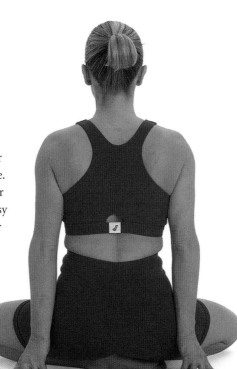

27 The Seated Spine Twist

Becoming Aware
Assume the Pole (page 17) but gently lean back, breathing slowly and deeply and feel yourself getting into the mood for today's pose. Take a last look at the personality traits (*gunas*). One of the purposes of hatha yoga (the yoga of balance) is to help you to restore the true balance of your character, so you find out what sort of person you are as you progress in your yoga.

Limbering
Perform Limber 6 (page 12).

Posture
Today's posture is the first version of the Seated Spine Twist (*ardha matsyendrasana*), sometimes known as the Preparatory Version of Matsyendra's Pose. Assume the Pole (page 17). Breathing quietly, lift your left foot, and place it on the floor outside your right knee. Sit up tall and check that your spine is vertical. Place your right hand behind you, palm flat and fingers pointing away from you. Don't turn your torso yet.

Lay your left palm on the outside of your left ankle. You will need to begin turning to do this. Continue to turn and look over your right shoulder. Before you settle into the pose, check that your spine is upright and that your rear hand is placed where it can give you the most support. Finally, check that your head has turned horizontally and has not developed a tilt.

Look out of the right-hand corners of your eyes. Settle in the pose, perhaps making little exhalations as you draw in your abdomen, and make room for a tiny little bit more rotation.

Don't rush. When you are ready, turn your head back first, so that you can see, and control the movements of your arms, legs and torso until you are back in the Pole.

Benefits
Rotations are complex movements, because everything in your torso changes position in relation to everything else. All your vertebrae move and all your muscles alternately give and take. All your internal organs get a healthy massage, and the *chakras* are stimulated. Performed carefully and regularly, this posture is a complete pick-me-up.

After a pause, with quiet breathing, perform on the other side. Then perform the two sides again.

Relaxation
Try lying face down again, and feel your joints and muscles 'easing out' after the work you have done with them today.

• Precautions
Rotations can have undesirable side-effects for people with neuro-muscular problems. If you have any doubts or you feel that something is wrong as soon as you begin Limber 6, change to the Lucky Pose (page 50).

Be aware of any discomfort in the rotations – this will be an indication that you have gone too far, too soon. It's good to pause thoughtfully in this posture, so pull back a little bit from the full turn so that you can hold a partial pose quietly without being distracted by the extremity of the pose.

28 The Dawn Horse

Becoming Aware

Assume the Pose of the Expert with the Gesture of Wisdom. Be attentive to the details of your pose, checking that you are stable and comfortable. Try a 4-4-4-4 breath in a more formal style. Inhale for 4 (*puraka*, expanding your body to attract breath and *prana*), hold the breath for 4 (*antar kumbhaka*, having a full 'pot' of air inside), exhale for 4 (*rechaka*, letting breath and *prana* flow out) and wait for 4 (*bahya kumbhaka*, having the 'pot' taken out).

Opening Energy Channels

Remain in the Pose of the Expert with the Gesture of Wisdom (or your chosen alternative) and perform Shining Skull (page 41). Today it will feel different, because you are performing it in the Pose of the Expert – your legs are open and your hands are out to the side. You may decide to use this base pose for Shining Skull in future because it enables the techniques to get to your abdomen better. Try making the pulses at two a second but keep them small. In time, work up to 50 pulses (25 seconds).

Breathing

Next perform the Cooling Breath (page 57). Close your eyes, and direct your awareness of the moving breath to your forehead. As you become familiar with the technique, try directing the breath to other places, especially where you have a problem.

The Seal of the Dawn Horse

Change to the Rock (page 16) for the Seal of the Dawn Horse or Riding the Horse at Dawn (*asvini*

mudra). If you have ever ridden a horse or stood up on your bike pedals, you will know the action involved in rising and falling in the stirrups. This posture asks you to make these movements.

Imagine you are riding a horse. Bump up and down, breathing easily. The 'ups' will need effort; the 'downs' will just happen. You will get out of breath at first, and you will also get warm. You may get a definite feeling that a 'ball of energy' has risen through you. Rest to let everything settle back into place.

Meditation

In your chosen pose – which can be the Rock – continue to observe the movements of *prana* but without moving your body. Become engrossed in this (*dharana*) and then quietly observe it continuing (*dhyana*).

Relaxation

Assume the Corpse (page 18) but with your legs quite widely apart and your arms a fair way from your body. This is the relaxation form of the Corpse. Feel calm, and enjoy today's relaxation. Imagine a hot summer's afternoon. Walk into a cool woodland glade and see the sunlight cascading down through the leaves, but don't form any thoughts; just enjoy it. Feel the cool air on your skin and notice all the fragrances of the moist woodland floor. Hear birdsong but don't wonder which birds are singing. As a light shower begins, catch a raindrop on your lips. Recall all these sensations together. Rest before concluding your programme.

29 More Rolling Around

Becoming Aware

Can you assume a formal Pole posture (page 17)? We are gradually phasing out the informal poses so that you can spend all your practice time on classic techniques. Be aware of your attention coming to rest on your performance of the Pole.

Limbering

Perform Limber 6 (page 12).

Breathing

Make sure your have plenty of space for today's programme, then assume the Corpse (page 18). See if you can introduce an 8-8-8-8 breath. Breathe fully out before you begin, and then inhale for 4 seconds in your abdomen, for 2 seconds more in your ribcage and for another 2 seconds in your chest. Your abdomen should swell slightly upwards, your ribcage should expand to each side, and your chest should move towards your chin. Hold the full breath for 8 seconds, and then exhale for 8 seconds, through the chest for 2, ribcage for 2 and abdomen for 4. Try to wait for 8 seconds before resting.

• Precautions

Today's asana is demanding, especially the lifting of the legs, and if you have spine problems keep to the easy version below.

＊ Adaptations

If this is too trying, explore a version where you lift one leg (or knee), with your hands under you head, and lower it to the mat over the other, straight, leg.

Turning the Abdomen Over

Today we will explore the full version of Turning the Abdomen Over (*jatara parivartanasana*), which we first met on page 52; if you have time, look at that again.

Assume the 'ready' version of the Corpse, with your legs together and your hands close to your body with palms down. Move your arms out to the side so they are level with your shoulders. Bend and lift your knees and straighten your legs so they are pointing to the ceiling. Inhale deeply. As you exhale, lower your legs to the floor on your right side. Let your left shoulder come up a bit if it needs to. Your legs should be parallel with your arms. Take a little time to correct the angles of your arms and legs. This will keep you in pose for a few moments, which will be good for you. The weight of your legs will help your body to rotate in a resting position.

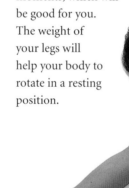

Prepare to inhale and as you do, lift your legs back to the top again. Don't worry if this is quite a struggle – you will become stronger soon.

Now perform all that on the other side. Start with the left side next time.

Relaxation

After this programme lie face down and let yourself 'melt down' into the floor.

Benefits
This exercise healthily extends your spine muscles and stimulates your internal organs.

30 The Half Lotus

Becoming Aware

It's time to explore the Lotus (*pad-masana*), the most important of the ancient seated postures. We will look at the easier version, the Half Lotus (*ardha padmasana*) or the Single-legged Lotus (*eka pad-masana*).

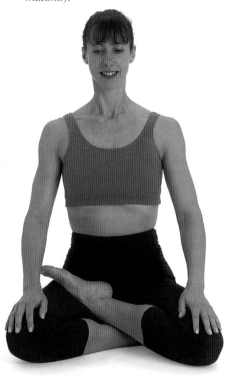

Begin as if you were going to assume the Pose of the Expert (page 22). Choose your best side and use two blocks if you need to. Fit your right (or left) heel well into your perineum, but have the knee less far to the side. Ease your left foot up onto the thigh of your right leg, and hold it in position, while you gently see if your left knee will lower onto the floor. If something hurts, stop at once and cuddle both your knees to ease them. If it works and you feel only a sensation of stiffness or fatigue, hold the pose for a few moments and then try the other side. If it all seems easy, use just one block or even none at all. Keep your hands free throughout to adjust your legs or keep them on your knees so that you don't fall backwards.

Opening Energy Channels

Perform Cleansing with Internal Fire (page 43).

Breathing

Next try assuming the Half Lotus for the Cooling Breath (page 57); if you prefer, stay in the Pose of the Expert.

Directing Inner Energy

We return to Homage. Assume the Rock. Can you make the Reverse Gesture of Greeting? If not, return your hands to the front. It's better to perform something that is within your present capa- 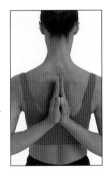 bilities and to do it well. Curl slowly down, letting your thoughts follow the movement, until your head touches the floor (or wherever you comfortably get to).

As you begin to uncurl, call to mind the *chakras* you visit along the way – at the base of your spine, in your pelvic area, at your navel, in your heart, at your neck, between your eyes and on the crown of your head. With care, you can time it so that each *chakra* opens as you pass it.

Now curl down again, closing the *chakras* as you go. Uncurl.

Meditation

Assume the Half Lotus or the Pose of the Expert with the Gesture of Wisdom and retrace the two pranic journeys you made in Homage, but without moving.

Relaxation

Today we will take a walk in the cool of an autumn evening. Remember that you should just 'be there'. Don't linger and start to form thoughts. Simply feel the sensations. Assume the relaxation version of the Corpse (page 61). Visit a country lane between trees. See late sunshine glinting through the autumn leaves and watch a brown leaf twirl as it falls to the leafy carpet beneath your feet. Hear rooks in a tall copse across the fields. Feel the softness of the leaves beneath your bare feet. Smell the fragrance of all the plants on the evening air and be rejuvenated by all these natural sensations.

See how rested you are. This is largely because your mind was engaged with its thoughts.

• Precautions

If you are not very supple, don't perse-vere with any of the advanced seated poses. Be patient, or you will hurt yourself. You will make most progress if you take little steps at a time.

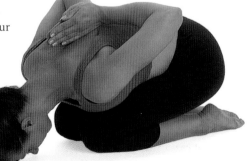

31 Sitting without a Chair

Benefits
A combination of the Powerful Pose and bottom shuffling is excellent for toning your buttocks and your thighs. Both exercises stimulate your blood circulation.

Becoming Aware

In a relaxed standing position and breathing gently, begin to assume the Mountain, but treat the movements as little rituals, requiring your full attention. Pay attention today to your body balances. Hatha yoga is the yoga of balance (*ha*, sun; *tha*, moon). You could use a mirror and see if you stand equally on your feet, equally on toes and heels and equally on the outside and inside edges of your feet.

Turn a little towards the mirror, and look at your vertical line. Are you 'straight up and down' or do you have a projecting bottom or abdomen or chest. Hatha yoga is about standing, kneeling, sitting and lying as truly balanced as possible.

Limbering
Perform Limber 4 (page 11).

Posture

Today's position is the Powerful Pose (*utkatasana*), which is sometimes also known as Sitting on an Imaginary Chair.

Assume the Mountain (page 15). Raise your arms until they are above your head, just behind your ears, but not touching them. Breathe quietly throughout. Lean forwards slightly and bend your knees, as if you were going to sit down. Stay in this half-leaning, half-sitting pose for a few moments if you can. It's about feeling balanced and strengthening your knees.

Carefully straighten up and lower your arms – and resume the Mountain. There is no reason why you can't perform this just in front

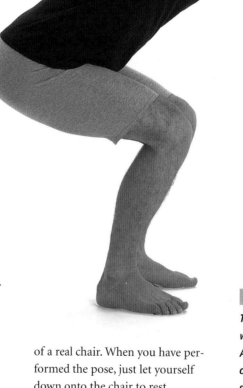

of a real chair. When you have performed the pose, just let yourself down onto the chair to rest. Perform it again by raising your arms and lifting yourself effortlessly off the chair.

Relaxation

After all that standing, sit down and cuddle your knees, rocking gently from side to side and 'stroke' all those muscles that you have used.

• Precautions

This is not suitable for people with weak or injured knees (see the Adaptations). If you are really concerned that your spine is not straight, see your doctor. Some faults are muscular and can probably be corrected, but you must always take the greatest care with your back and neck.

* Adaptations

Sit down in the Pole (page 17). Raise your arms and use all your body muscles to help you to shuffle forwards on your buttocks – and then shuffle back.

32 Piercing the Sun

Becoming Aware

Assume the Pose of the Expert with your hands in the Gesture of Wisdom or, if you can do it without discomfort, the Half Lotus (page 63) and be quiet for a few moments.

Opening Energy Channels

In your chosen pose, perform Alternate Nostril Breathing (page 35). Sit tall, and try for a 6-6-6-6 pattern of breathing (in for 6, hold for 6, out for 6 and wait for 6 seconds). Having a second pulse during your practice is becoming increasingly important.

Breathing

Today we begin to practise Piercing the Sun (*surya bedha*), breathing in through the right nostril.

Assume the Rock with your hands flat on the tops of your thighs. If kneeling is difficult, use a stool so that your body weight is not on your feet. Using your right hand, lay the middle finger on your left nostril, and breathe in through your right nostril (feel that you are taking in *prana* as well). Hold the breath (and the *prana*) – you can put your hand back on your thigh. Now lay that same middle finger on your right nostril, and let out your breath (and some *prana*) through your left nostril. Finally, hold yourself empty of breath and *prana*. Put your hand back on your thigh and rest. That is one round of Piercing the Sun; we will continue to explore this technique on page 67.

Directing Inner Energy

If you can, assume either the Half Lotus (page 63) with the Gesture of Wisdom or the Pose of the Expert with the Gesture of Wisdom, and remain in that pose for meditation. Remember to use both sides of your body alternately, so that you can be sure that you are developing a true sense of yogic balance.

Perform the Space-walker (page 47). Turn your tongue back inside your mouth so that it sits in the sinus hollow at the back of your upper palate. Breathe quietly. The idea is to focus your mind on what the position feels like and so encourage *prana* to gather there and energize your sinuses. Hold the position and then rest.

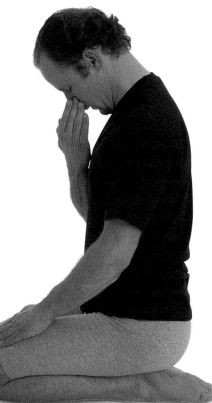

Meditation

Make sure that your pose is comfortable, altering it if you wish. Let your thoughts settle on your root energy centre (*muladhara chakra*). Become aware of the physical sensation of sitting on your tail-bone. Adjust your pose if you can't feel it. Your root energy centre is at the base of your spine. You have opened it and will begin to feel grounded and stable.

In yoga tradition, this *chakra* has a rich symbolism. See if you can picture, in your mind's eye, a circle of *prana* with four petals (representing earth, air, fire and water) and a glowing red colour.

An open root energy centre will help to look after the health of your lower body, especially your legs. Let your mind dwell quietly on the *chakra*, so that it gently closes down again.

Relaxation

Assume the Corpse, then imagine that you are going to get wrapped up warm for a short walk in the snow. Feel the snow falling on your cheeks. See the soft snow lying on tops of the hedges. Hear your own footsteps crunching as you go. Then go indoors and feel the warm and enjoy the taste of your favourite hot drink. Feel drowsy, and fall asleep in front of the log fire – but wake up again, because your practice is over.

✳ Adaptations

If you have problems with chakras, remember that they correspond to nerve centres. In this programme you have been concentrating on your sacral plexus.

33 The Child

Becoming Aware

Assume a formal Pole position. Be attentive to the way the pose feels, especially when you have completed it and are still. That stillness, of mind as well as of body, is the direct result of the care you took to assume the pose. The pose itself and completing it with a breath, is very much what hatha yoga is about, but the stillness is a central feature of raja yoga (royal yoga). You regularly perform the three special techniques of raja yoga: concentration (*dharana*), contemplation (*dhyana*) and spiritual freedom (*samadhi*), but we call them all by the general name of meditation (*samyama*).

Limbering

Perform Limber 2 (page 10).

Posture

Today's posture, the Child (*susukhasana*), is sometimes performed as a relaxation or as a rest between poses. We are going to give it full *asana* status.

Assume the Rock (page 16). Let your arms rest beside you, the backs of the hands towards, or on, the floor, and fingers pointing to the rear. Resist the temptation to move your hands as you complete this posture – you will find that they are in the right place all the way through.

Curl forwards, starting with your head, and breathing gently. Curl down until your head touches the mat.

Finally, let your elbows bend out slightly and come to the floor. This completes the pose known as the Soft Child, but if you wish, you can turn your head to the side as you exhale, to the centre again as you inhale and to the other side as you exhale. You may find that you can perform this pose without lifting your bottom from your heels. If it has popped up, don't worry – but don't adjust anything, to get it down. Uncurl in the reverse order, keeping your hands in position and making a deeper inhalation as you come to the top of the pose.

The Strong Child pose is the same, except that you don't curl down. Keep your back flat and open your chest. Draw your shoulders back so that you actually lunge down. This creates pressure between your chest and your thighs – feel this pressure making you exhale. On the way up, lift your head first, draw your shoulders back and flatten your back, inhaling as you reach the top.

After you have performed this pose you need to move your body in the opposite direction and rest in the new position for about 12 seconds.

Relaxation

Let your body tell you how it wants to relax. You can, if you have time, go straight on to the next programme, in which case omit this Relaxation and the time spent on becoming aware in the second programme and proceed with Candle Gazing.

• Precautions

There are no dangers with this programme, but you should be careful not to have your head too low if you have heart problems.

34 The Essential You

Becoming Aware

You are now familiar with several seated poses and may prefer to make your own choice of a pose for the techniques in this programme. Choose poses that are just within your ability, so that you make regular progress, but choose ones that are comfortable for times when you want to stay in a pose for quite a while. Select a pose now that you can keep for a few moments, to get focused, and go on to use again for Candle Gazing.

Opening Energy Channels

Perform Candle Gazing (page 37). Feel more deeply the meditative aspects of this technique. Not only are you cleansing your eyes, and your sinuses, but you are also opening the energy channels in your head.

Breathing

Today we will look at two new aspects of Piercing the Sun. Assume a kneeling pose, but remember to kneel really tall. First, the recommended breathing counts (have a second pulse handy; most electronic clocks have one): exhale deeply, without a special count; now inhale for 6, hold for 18, exhale for 8, and wait for 4. If this is difficult, make a note to work at it, and for the time being make the counts 4-12-6-2. Rest after each attempt. Don't perform more than four rounds.

Now we will look at the locks (*bandhas*). Breathing quietly, apply Root Lock (*mulabandha*) by tightening the muscles in your perineum (pelvic floor) – it's like trying to bring your front and rear openings

closer together. Release again and perform once or twice more, trying to make the movement definite, without being violent.

Now perform the Waterpipe Lock (*jalamdhara bandha*). Tilt your head back a little, then tilt it forwards at the very top of your neck, as if you were trying to see something on your neck. Your chest will lift if you do this properly, so you will want to inhale. Lift your head back, again at the top of your neck, and tilt it slightly back so that you can tilt it forwards from your shoulders, back into place. Exhale. Do this once or twice more.

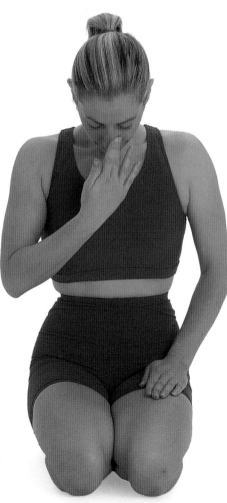

Directing Inner Energy

Assume the Pole and perform the Seal of the Container (page 49).

Meditation

Choose a seated pose that is comfortable and in which your thighs and knees open. Sit tall and focus on the energy centre in your pelvic area (*svadisthana chakra*). This is the 'sweet centre of personal energy'. As you sit, imagine an orange glow around your hips and a flower with six petals circling an ocean of energy. Focusing on it is enough to open it, and you will already be gaining emotional energy and strength. If you have kidney or bladder problems, open the *chakra* and focus on it. Sit quietly, focusing on the *chakra*, and end by gently fading out the orange glow and putting the *chakra* back to rest.

Relaxation

Lie in the full Corpse position and imagine that you are lying under a shady tree in a beautiful garden, with strong sunlight filtering through the leaves. Feel a shaft of really warm sunlight resting on your left foot, and as the leaves move in the light breeze, feel it moving up to your ankle and shin, and back again. As you lie in this paradise, feel the sunspot move up to your knee and to your thigh, and back to your shin.

Finally, feel it settle on your thigh and sense the warmth sinking deeply down into your body so that it is carried by your circulation to every part of you. Have a little stretch before you get up and turn on one side to make getting up a bit easier.

35 The Full Seated Spine Twist

Benefits
Rotations imitate the *chakras* and stimulate energy, so you should begin to feel wonderful. But just as we need to close the *chakras* before concluding our practice, it's vital that you always rotate in both directions – and remember to alternate the side you start with.

Becoming Aware

Bring some of the skills you have learned in meditation and contemplation programmes into your practice, and assume the Easy Pose with the Gesture of Knowledge. This will underline for you the role that hatha yoga plays in preparing you for raja yoga. As you make the body shape of the Easy Pose, concentrate on the movements you make with your legs, arms and hands. Settle down for a few quiet moments before you go on to the limbering.

Limbering

Perform Limber 6 (page 12).

Posture

We have already looked at the Seated Spine Twist (page 60), and today we will perform the Full Seated Spine Twist (*ardha matsyendrasana*). Assume the Pole (page 17) and bring your left foot up beside your right knee. You need only one hand for this, so use the other one on the floor beside you to keep your spine tall. Now use both hands to lift the foot over to the outside of your right knee. Here is a major difference from the earlier version. Lift your right arm up and over your left knee and lay the palm of the hand on the side of your left thigh, taking your left hand behind you to support your spine. Turn your head to the left and look behind you. Breathe quietly through all this and, maintaining the pose, close your eyes and feel the way you have rotated your body twice – the lower body to the right, and the upper body to the left. The inner energy channels (*nadis*) are believed to spiral like this, so you are in a state of total revolution.

As before, turn your head back first, so that you can keep your eye on how you bring the rest of you back to the front. Don't forget to resume a good Pole position, before repeating the pose on the other side.

Relaxation

Lie down and cuddle your knees, rocking a little to and fro or from side to side. This will let your spine open and lengthen, easing out any stiffness. If you don't do this, you may find that you are stiff later on.

• Precautions

Do not attempt the full pose if you suffer from conditions such as arthritis, some nervous disorders, low blood pressure or dizziness. However, a little gentle work with the easy version should be safe and will softly exercise your spine. If you like, omit the head movements.

36 City of Jewels

Benefits
Asthmatics will benefit
enormously from controlled
breathing techniques.

Becoming Aware

Choose a seated pose and spend a few moments withdrawing from your daily world and waking up to the inner world of your real self.

Opening Energy Channels

Next, assume a seated pose in which you are comfortable and perform Head-furrow Cleansing (page 39). Be relaxed and slow, relishing the sensations.

Breathing

Today we are going to continue our exploration of Piercing the Sun, this time with the Lock that Flies Up (page 39). First, perform two or three deep but gentle breaths, to set the *prana* in motion. Now take a deep breath in. Pause, then breathe powerfully out and wait for a few moments before resting. Do this again and as you exhale, draw your abdomen back towards your spine and up under your ribs. The movement will add to the power of the exhalation. Keep your lungs empty with your abdomen still pulled up and back. This is the Lock that Flies Up, a muscle movement that causes your abdomen to 'jump up' and concentrates *prana* in your lower body.

Try to release the lock without releasing the breath. Then exhale. Perform the lock once more, but with the middle finger of your right hand closing your left nostril. Count 8 seconds, from beginning to breathing out. Don't over-breathe – you could damage your diaphragm or get dizzy or both.

Directing Inner Energy

Today, repeat the *mudra* Looking at the Void (page 51). You will still be in the learning stage, so be gentle but persistent.

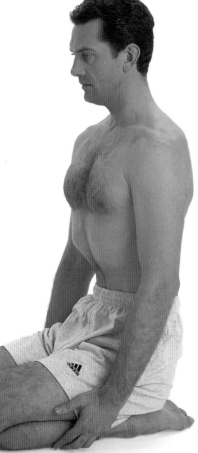

• **Precautions**

If you are pregnant do not try holding your breath, either in or out.

Meditation

If you are quite comfortable, stay in your pose. Otherwise, change to another seated pose or change your legs over. Sit tall, inhale deeply into your chest and exhale into your abdomen – a kind of gentle Lock that Flies Up. Now go on breathing in your abdomen only, keeping your chest lifted and wide.

As you move your navel forwards and back, become aware of the pranic or astral centre (*manipura chakra*) in your central pranic channel (*sushumna nadi*) in your spine and level with your navel. This *chakra* is all about feelings – we often seem to get feelings in our stomachs – and it's also to do with the digestive system. There is a special *prana*, the astral current (*samana vayu*) that works in that area. For now, though, just sit with your navel moving gently.

Relaxation

Try relaxing on your front today. Lie quietly in a comfortable position and imagine the sun shining through leafy branches, so that you can feel its rays on the backs of your legs, perhaps starting on your calves, then moving with the breeze to the backs of your knees and eventually onto the backs of your thighs. Just feel the sun's rays – don't let thoughts get in the way of the pleasure!

✳ **Adaptations**

If holding your breath is not for you, just go on breathing calmly. But don't over-breathe.

37 The Supported Shoulder Stand

Becoming Aware

Glance back at page 68 and assume the Easy Pose with the Gesture of Knowledge but with your legs the other way around.

Spend some time thinking about karma yoga (the yoga of action), in which kind actions, thoughts and words bring you many physical, mental, emotional and spiritual benefits. Karma yoga works best when those actions just 'happen' rather than when you are really thinking about the benefits.

Limbering

Perform Limber 8 (page 12).

Posture

We are going to perform the Supported Shoulder Stand (*salambha sarvangasana*). Breathe quietly throughout, unless we suggest otherwise, but don't forget to breathe.

Begin by assuming the Corpse (page 18). Bring your knees up to your chest and then use your arms to help bring them up onto your forehead, placing your hands on your spine to support you. If you can't manage this, try sitting with your knees against chest and letting yourself tumble back so that your legs move up and over into the same position.

The secret of this posture is to make sure that you are actually standing on your shoulder tops. You can do this by easing your shoulder tops out, using your arms to help you. When you feel that your back is vertical, begin to straighten your legs, raising your feet towards the ceiling while keeping your feet flat. Stay in the pose for a few moments, breathing gently.

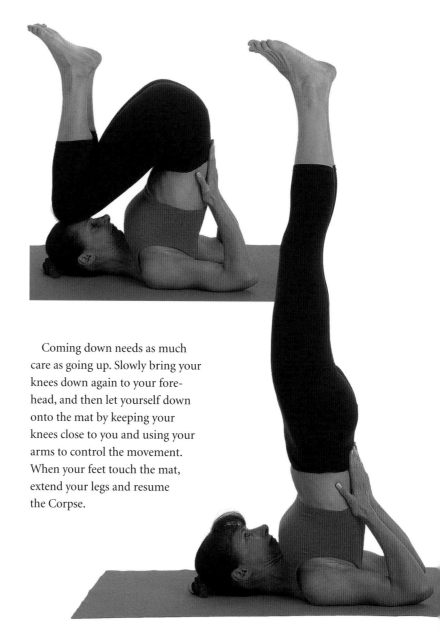

Coming down needs as much care as going up. Slowly bring your knees down again to your forehead, and then let yourself down onto the mat by keeping your knees close to you and using your arms to control the movement. When your feet touch the mat, extend your legs and resume the Corpse.

After you have performed this pose you need to move your body in the opposite direction and rest in the new position for about 12 seconds.

Relaxation

Lie face down, as a rest from the Corpse, and 'melt' into the floor.

• Precautions

You must not attempt inverted postures if you are pregnant, have a hernia, abnormal blood pressure, a detached retina or heart problems. Today's posture is not suitable for anyone who needs to avoid having their torso upside down. The Boat (page 42) is a good alternative.

38 An Affair of the Heart

Becoming Aware
Choose a kneeling pose that you can maintain throughout today's programme. Be still and become aware of the calm.

Opening Energy Channels
Perform Shining Skull (page 41), keeping your abdominal movements small and regular. You are going to practise Piercing the Sun shortly, so emphasize the difference.

Breathing
You have learned all the parts of Piercing the Sun, and now we will put them together. Keep in mind that the high point of the exercise is breathing in air and *prana* through the right nostril (*puraka* through the *pingala nadi*).

Make sure you are comfortable in the kneeling pose you have chosen and gently breathe fully out. Inhale through the right nostril for 6 seconds, then apply the Root Lock (page 35) and the Waterpipe Lock (page 37). Hold the breath for 12; release the Waterpipe Lock and then the Root Lock.

Exhale through the left nostril, making the Lock that Flies Up (page 39) for 8 seconds. Release the lock and return to quiet breathing.

Directing Inner Energy
Try to hold the same pose. You should be beginning to feel a steady level of awareness flowing through you – try not to interrupt the flow. Perform the Seal of Shiva (page 53), but if you feel it is still unfamiliar, take it slowly. To conclude, either come down again in steps or just close your eyes. Alternatively, just gaze at the tip of your nose: this is *nasikagra mudra*.

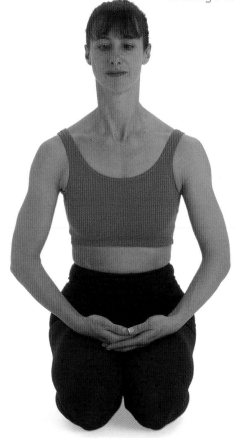

Lord Krishna says to Arjuna, his devotee: 'Listen again to this: it's my most special message to you, and full of mystery: "I love you very much".'
Bhagavad Gita 18:64

Meditation
Change your pose to one that is comfortable but make sure you are sitting tall. Look inside your heart and listen to your heartbeat. The *chakra* is all about love (naturally) but also to do with your lungs and circulation and the health of your upper torso. Just below the inner energy centre of the heart (*anahata chakra*) is the wishing or kalpa tree. When you have opened your energy centre, you can make wishes: 'I wish, with all my heart ...'

Sit quietly and feel loved. Feel the love you have for your family and your friends. Then just sit, without feeling any need to think at all. If thoughts start tumbling into your head, simply watch them tumble out again. If you like, imagine a green mist surrounding that part of you. Remember to close both *chakras* at the end of your meditation period.

Relaxation
Adopt any pose that is comfortable and think about sunshine again. Feel rays of strong sunshine passing over your hands and along your forearms and back again.

39 The Unsupported Shoulder Stand

Becoming Aware

Assume the Pose of the Expert with your hands in the Gesture of Consciousness. Settle and feel good about having this time to yourself.

Limbering

Perform Limber 8 (page 12).

Posture

Today's posture, the Unsupported Shoulder Stand (*niralamba sarvangasana*), begins from the full supported version (page 70), so that's where we'll start.

Assume the Corpse (page 18), but with your legs together and your arms beside you, palms down. Inhale. Exhale and bend your knees, first to your chest, and then, by pressing down with your arms and flexing your abdominal muscles, bring your knees to your forehead.

Place your hands flat on your spine to support you while you ease out your shoulder tops. Move your spine up until it is well on the way to being vertical. Breathe gently now. Keep your hands in place while you slowly straighten your legs. Keep your feet flat to the ceiling. Pause in the pose, so that your body and mind can obtain the benefits. If you feel that you should conclude the pose now, omit the next paragraph.

If you are comfortable in the pose, move your legs slightly to the rear and feel your spine move a little way away from your hands. When that happens, carefully place your hands on the sides of your thighs so that you are balanced on your shoulder tops and your shoulder stand is unsupported. To return to the supported pose, put your hands back on your spine, but move carefully so that you do not lose your balance.

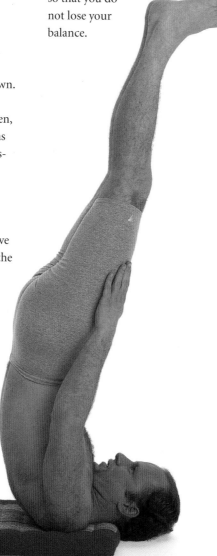

Benefits
The pose causes major changes in the patterns of blood pressure. There is less pressure in the legs, making them feel enormously refreshed, and more in the brain, giving a feeling of increased alertness. All your internal organs will be stimulated by being moved around in relation to gravity and to each other.

To conclude the pose, bend your knees and bring them back down to your forehead and put your hands back on the mat. Keeping your legs folded close to your chest, slowly roll down to the mat. Let your head pop up, but let it down again by cuddling your knees. Assume the resting version of the Corpse, with your legs apart and your arms away from your body, palms up, and lie quietly, breathing as you need. If you feel able, perform both poses again.

After you have performed this pose you need to move your body in the opposite direction and rest there for about 12 seconds.

Relaxation

Continue relaxing in the Corpse.

• Precautions

If you have to avoid inversions, shoulder stands are not for you. Try the Boat (page 42) instead. If you are in good health, these poses are perfectly safe, provided that you take our advice seriously. Do not perform if your neck starts to hurt and always come down slowly, as we have shown you.

✴ Adaptations

Do try using a cushion under your shoulders; it could protect you from a damaged neck.

40 The Pure Energy Centre

Becoming Aware

Select a classical pose and sit still. It's a good idea to move through the poses we are exploring – the Easy Pose, the Pose of the Expert, the Half Lotus and the Lotus. Always explore the ones you can only just do! Don't forget to alternate your legs. And experiment with different gestures, perhaps moving through the series on page 24.

Opening Energy Channels

Assume the Rock for Cleansing with Internal Fire (page 43). In this pose you will feel the effect of the techniques on your lower spine and your root energy centre will be opened.

Breathing

Next, still in the Rock, perform Piercing the Sun (page 65) twice. First, perform slowly, paying attention to each movement and then perform with your eyes closed, and just let it happen. Don't worry if you forget something or get the counting wrong – you can go on learning and experimenting by choosing Piercing the Sun in your personal selection of techniques later on.

Directing Inner Energy

Today we're going to explore the Seal of the Six Openings (page 55) again, but this time in the Rock. You will have to relearn all the details, but that's all right, because yoga is all about attention to detail. The more familiar you are with it, the more clearly you will hear your inner body sounds, and the subtle sounds of *prana* in the *nadis*. Notice again how refreshed your senses are when you return to the Rock.

Two birds are sitting on the same tree; One is eating the fruit; the other just sits, looking on.
Mundaka Upanishad III:1:1

Meditation

Assume a seated pose and with your hands in the gesture of your choice. Complete the pose with a slow, deep inhalation into your upper chest and a careful exhalation in your abdomen. Remain sitting tall. Try to perform still breathing (page 47) in your abdomen only during your meditation. Think about the soft skin where your neck meets your chest. Just behind that spot, in your central energy channel (*sushumna*), is the essentially pure astral centre (*visuddha chakra*). Sometimes called the Treasury of Sound, it's really all about the way we communicate. Therefore, a good way to feel confident about talking to people, to be alive to other people's body language and to cure a sore throat, is to work with *visuddha chakra*. Meditate on it and perform techniques that include the Waterpipe Lock (page 37) or even doing the lock on its own.

Relaxation

As your period of meditation grows in duration and in importance in your practice, you will find that you only need a few moments resting, and you may not even wish to lie down. Simply relaxing in your seated pose and perhaps reading something soothing, will rest your body and mind and close your *chakras*. Remember to feel the sun on your arms again – perhaps on the backs of your arms, where the skin is softer and more receptive.

✳ Adaptations

The best alternative to strong abdomen movements is little ones.

41 The First Dancer

Becoming Aware

Assume a seated pose. It's only for a few moments, so try one that you can only just do. The idea in yoga is that you always move onwards, extending your natural physical limits and expanding your mental and spiritual horizons. The fourth main classical yoga is bhakti yoga (the yoga of devotion).

How can being devoted to a god or a revered teacher or a hero of your imagination be yogic? If yoga is a way of finding wholeness and balance, then in hatha and raja yoga we do this by postures, breathing and meditation. In karma yoga we do it by taking opportunities to help other people. In bhakti yoga, in the act and deep experience of devotion, we discover wholeness, fulfilment and bliss. The devotion must be simple, free and uncomplicated – totally without ulterior motive.

Limbering

Perform Limber 1 (page 9).

Posture

Today's posture is the first version of the Dancer (*natarajasana*).

Begin by assuming the Mountain (page 15). Are you balanced? Can you stay comfortably in the Mountain with your eyes closed? That will be a good preparation for today's pose. If balancing is not your strong point, rest your spare hand on a chairback as we go along. Breathe gently throughout.

Stand tall. Raise your left knee towards your chest. Cup your left hand around that left foot and take the foot under you to the rear. Hold it gently in position, with the heel near your left buttock.

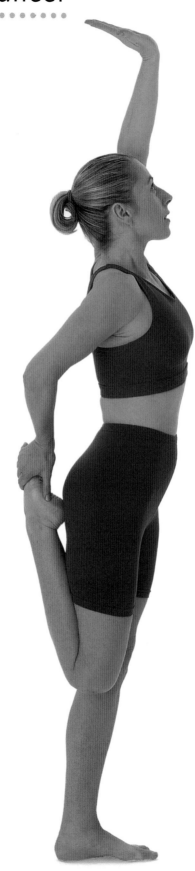

Raise your right arm until it is beside your right ear. Reach up and turn your palm flat to the ceiling. Looking straight ahead, lift your chest. You are the Dancer.

To return, lower your right arm first, then your left foot and finally your left arm. Resume the Mountain.

Now perform it on the other side, using a chair again if necessary. Start on the right side this time, taking your right foot under you and not to the side. This time, pull your heel in behind you until you can feel it making a dent in your buttock. Raise your left arm straight and strong from the shoulder. If you are contented in the pose, try closing your eyes for a moment.

Balanced poses are among the high points of yoga, because they need suppleness, stamina and balance. You can do them best if you are quite relaxed.

Relaxation

Be still for a few moments.

＊ Adaptations

You can perform the Dancer in two halves – the standing part only and the upper arm separately.

74

42 The Third Eye Again

Becoming Aware
Sit relaxed and still in the Easy Pose with your hands in the Gesture of Knowledge.

Breathing
Stay in position and perform several rounds of Alternate Nostril Breathing (page 35). Pay attention to your movements, watching the energy ways open and fill.

The Bee Breath
Next, we are going to look at a new technique, the Bee Breath (*bhramari*). Assume the Rock (page 16) and practise humming. Inhale deeply and, as you exhale, hum softly, gradually getting louder, then quieter again until you fade out. Exhale completely. As you inhale, hum softly, gradually getting louder and then quieter again, until you fade out. Repeat this exercise, but go for a low note as you breathe out and a high note as you breathe in. Humming makes you breathe slowly, which is good for you, but the vibrations will stimulate astral energy (*prana*) – the low note in your chest and the high note in your head. If you have time, try the two hums again.

Directing Inner Energy
Sit in the Pole (page 17) and perform the Great Seal (page 57). Be sure to hold the breath full in the final positions.

Meditation
Sit tall in your chosen pose. Centre your thoughts on your forehead, in the centre – just above your nose. Use your hands to help you, if you like. Just inside is your 'command centre' (*ajna chakra*) or third eye.

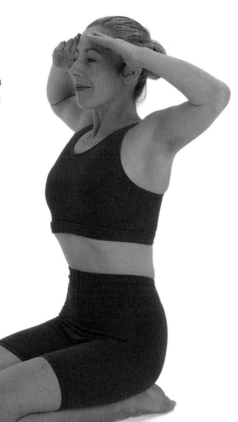

Benefits
Humming is a good introduction to chanting (*mantra*). Physical vibrations can improve muscle tone, stimulate the circulation and cleanse the sinuses.

See an indigo glow surrounding your head and feel yourself becoming tremendously alert. This *chakra* takes care of your head and all its contents – your face (eyes, nose, ears, mouth, sinuses) and your brain and main nerve centre. Sit tall and enjoy the indigo glow and feel happy.

Relaxation
Assume the Prone Corpse (page 19) and imagine that you are lying on your favourite beach. Soak up the sun as it warms your shoulders. Feel the effect as a cloud obscures the sun and passes over. Feel the warmth returns. Make sure you are fully awake before you get up.

• Precautions
Go carefully with the Great Seal if you are pregnant.

Signs of progress in hatha yoga are a clear complexion, very clear eyes, good health, active digestion and open energy channels.
Hathayoga Pradipika 2:77–8

43 The Gateway

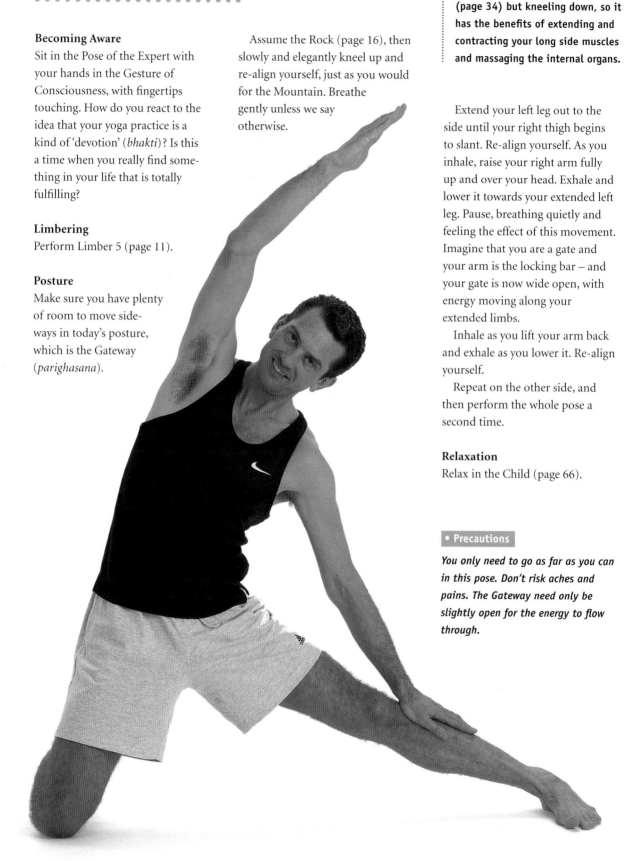

Becoming Aware

Sit in the Pose of the Expert with your hands in the Gesture of Consciousness, with fingertips touching. How do you react to the idea that your yoga practice is a kind of 'devotion' (*bhakti*)? Is this a time when you really find something in your life that is totally fulfilling?

Limbering

Perform Limber 5 (page 11).

Posture

Make sure you have plenty of room to move sideways in today's posture, which is the Gateway (*parighasana*).

Assume the Rock (page 16), then slowly and elegantly kneel up and re-align yourself, just as you would for the Mountain. Breathe gently unless we say otherwise.

Benefits

This pose is just like the Moon (page 34) but kneeling down, so it has the benefits of extending and contracting your long side muscles and massaging the internal organs.

Extend your left leg out to the side until your right thigh begins to slant. Re-align yourself. As you inhale, raise your right arm fully up and over your head. Exhale and lower it towards your extended left leg. Pause, breathing quietly and feeling the effect of this movement. Imagine that you are a gate and your arm is the locking bar – and your gate is now wide open, with energy moving along your extended limbs.

Inhale as you lift your arm back and exhale as you lower it. Re-align yourself.

Repeat on the other side, and then perform the whole pose a second time.

Relaxation

Relax in the Child (page 66).

• Precautions

You only need to go as far as you can in this pose. Don't risk aches and pains. The Gateway need only be slightly open for the energy to flow through.

44 The Coronet of Violets

Becoming Aware

Choose a seated pose for Candle Gazing and be quiet and still.

Opening Energy Channels

Perform Candle Gazing (page 37), becoming wide-eyed and open-minded.

Breathing

Today we will work with the Bee Breath (page 75) again. Kneel in the Rock and perform two rounds of the Complete Yoga Breath (page 35). Now inhale deeply with a high-pitched hum. Exhale with a low-pitched hum. Repeat. Put your thumbs in your ears and do it all again. Notice how the sound is now inside you. Rest, and do it again. Pause at the end of each hum, to let it resound, and move your energy around. Finally, perform one more round, making the hums as long as you can.

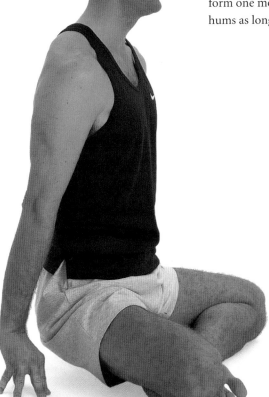

Directing Inner Energy

Now we will look again at the Big Poker (page 59). Assume the Easy Pose with your palms pressed down onto the floor. Inhale strongly and push yourself up off the floor or the block. Then make a sudden, strong exhalation and let yourself bump back down. The Big Poker is superb for toning the buttocks, but it will also give your astral energy a real boost. Perform it a couple more times.

Meditation

Settle into a pose of your choice, sit tall and take a deep breath. Imagine you are seated on the crown of your head inside a coronet of violet flowers. You are also inside the thousand-petalled lotus flower that crowns your innermost personal energy (*sahasrara chakra*). As your thoughts dwell on this centre, say your name and then say: 'I matter.' You may find this hard to do – many people do – but persevere. You don't have to be a shrinking violet when you are doing yoga.

Relaxation

Why not rest today just as you are and imagine that rays of warm sunshine are playing over your shoulders and your head. Wait for the sun to go in and for your *chakra* to close before you get up.

• Precautions

Do not perform Candle Gazing if you have eye problems or any nervous disorders.

✱ Adaptations

You can gaze at the candle with your eyes closed!

45 Going West

Benefits
This pose extends your spine and massages your chest and abdomen, while you just sit and watch.

Becoming Aware
Assume the Pose of the Expert if you can, with your hands in the Second Gesture of Consciousness and look forward to exploring one of the most distinguished poses in yoga. Pause to consider how you relate to your world.

Limbering
Perform Limber 3 (page 10).

Posture
Today's posture is the Seated Forward Bend (*paschimot-tanasana*), which is also known as Extending your Western Side.

Assume the Pole (page 17) and raise your arms forwards and up above your head, inhaling as you do.

Exhale and fold your spine down, from your hips, until your arms come to rest on the mat – it doesn't matter where. Now wait at least 20 seconds for your back to respond to that movement and for the muscles to lengthen. You are 'extending your western side' – that is, your back.

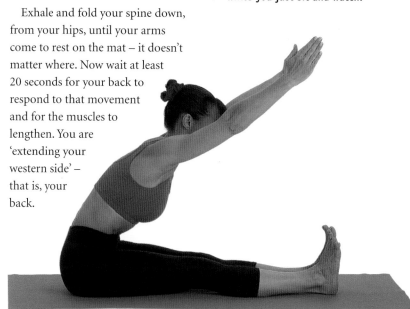

If all is well, take another breath and fold down a little further, maybe getting your chest to lie on your thighs. If you can, cup your first fingers around your big toes and rest your head on your knees.

If this is too difficult, do it a different way. From the Pole, raise your knees and rest your chest on your thighs. Now, with quiet breathing, let your knees down again, little by little, but keeping your chest in contact. Stop when your chest no longer makes contact.

Whichever way you choose, come up again, your hands moving back along the mat, until you can inhale yourself up into the Pole again. Now do it all again; but remember to balance at the end.

Relaxation
Rest in the Corpse for a nice passive relaxation.

• Precautions

Do listen to your back in this posture and make sure you distinguish between stiffness and pain.

46 Bees and Horses

Becoming Aware
Select a meditation pose you like and sit tall while you complete at least two rounds of the Complete Yoga Breath (page 35).

Opening Energy Channels
Stay in your position for Head-furrow Cleansing (page 39). Spend some time on this – every stroke of your thumb will ease out the tensions that inhibit energy flow.

Breathing
Today we will be looking at the Bee Breath again (page 75). Be aware that in the ancient yoga tradition, the in-breath hum is the tiny male bee, and the out-breath hum is the enormous queen bee. Perform one round to see how you are getting on with it.

Now perfect your seated pose. Put your thumbs in your ears, letting your fingers rest on your temples, so that you feel comfortable and your hands make a special kind of gesture. Pause. After breathing fully out, inhale, humming high, for 6 seconds. Pause again, but this time for 6 seconds. Exhale, humming low, for 6 seconds, and finish with a 6-second pause.

Perform again, being aware of the vibrations. Do you feel the high tones in your third eye (*ajna chakra*)? Do you feel the low ones in your heart centre (*anahata chakra*)? They'll be there, stimulating energy.

Directing Inner Energy
Do you remember the Seal of the Dawn Horse (page 61)? Can you bounce in this pose? Change if you want to – the Rock is a good one for horses. Imagine you are riding the horse at dawn, maybe through the

When astral energy fills the central astral channel … The mind will be still.
Hathayoga Pradipika 3:3

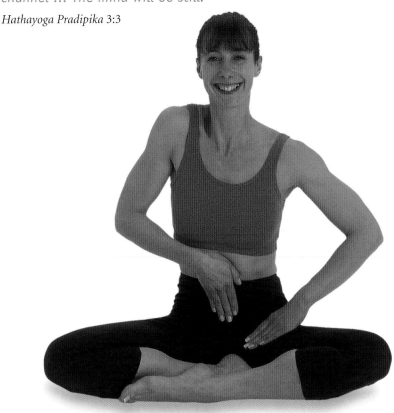

waves where the sea pounds the beach. Every lift makes a space for the energy and every bounce sends it tearing round your energy power-house (*kanda*) around your hips.

Meditation
Calm down again and choose your best pose for today's meditation. Try taking your awareness first to your root centre (*muladhara chakra*) and from there to your pelvic centre (*svadisthana chakra*). It's good to follow the energy through two or more centres – you can use your hands. The journey from root to pelvis isn't easy – yogic tradition believes that there is a 'block' between the two, making

transfer difficult. There is a solution – the root centre is a gathering of basic physical ideas, and the pelvic centre of emotional events. As you take your awareness up to your pubic centre, think of all its associations as emotional rather than physical, and you will succeed.

Relaxation
If you would prefer to lie down, lie face down so that you can feel the sun's rays on your shoulder blades and the back of your neck.

> ● **Precautions**
>
> **Don't do the Seal of the Dawn Horse with liquid in your stomach.**

Building Bridges

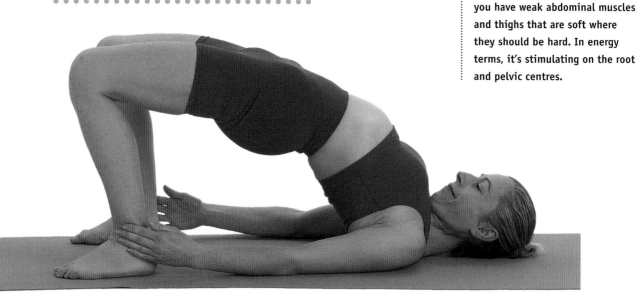

Benefits
The Bridge is especially good if you have weak abdominal muscles and thighs that are soft where they should be hard. In energy terms, it's stimulating on the root and pelvic centres.

Becoming Aware

Become quiet and still and consider the first of the five moral values (*yamas*) recommended by yoga teaching, total harmlessness (*ahimsa*). The idea is that we should not only avoid hurting each other or anything around us, but that we should not even allow hurtful thoughts to occupy our minds and certainly not let them find expression in words. Yoga would also add that we should not be violent to ourselves in any way in our practice.

Limbering

Perform Limber 3 (page 10).

Posture

Today's posture is the Bridge (*setu bandha*), which raises the spine from floor level into an arch. It has the advantage that you can lift all the way, or only a little way, or in between, and all the movements are useful.

Begin by assuming the Corpse (page 18). Breathing quietly, bend your knees. Can you touch your heels? Can you grasp your heels? You might manage it if you tuck your shoulders under you or if you go for one heel at a time. If you cannot do this, ignore the rest of this paragraph. If you can grasp your heels, do so. Now begin to lift your spine, starting with your tail-bone – which you should curl up and away from the mat. Let the lifting continue, bone by bone, up your spine, until your neck lifts away from the mat. Push down on your feet and press your shoulders under you to get a full lifting movement. You may find that your thighs are horizontal, like a table, and this is a sign that you have made the full movement. Apart from toning your thigh and abdominal muscles, this pose opens your root, pelvic, navel and heart *chakras*.

It's perfectly all right to lift without grasping your heels. You will need more power in your thighs and abdomen, and you may feel that your feet are slipping away from you. You can buy non-slip mats, but remember that there are times in yoga practice when you need to slip a little.

Whichever method you adopt, take care to come down in precisely the reverse order. Release your shoulders carefully, and then put one vertebra back on the mat at a time, tucking your tail-bone under as you complete the movement. Perform again, while the memory is still fresh.

After you have performed this pose you need to move your body in the opposite direction and rest in the new position for about 12 seconds.

Relaxation

Try relaxing on your side, curled up small and warm.

• Precautions

You should think twice about the Bridge if you have neck problems.

✻ Adaptations

Shoulder stretches in the Pole (see page 42) are a good alternative, and can be demanding, so be careful.

48 Energetic Journeys

Becoming Aware
Kneel in the Rock (page 16), breathe gently and feel calm. Rock gently to and fro.

Opening Energy Channels
Stay in the Rock and perform Cleansing with Internal Fire (page 43).

Breathing
Perform the Bee Breath (page 75) twice, the first time to recall the details and then just to enjoy it. Let the pauses last and last, so that you can feel the vibrations and benefit from them.

Directing Inner Energy
Stay in the Rock to perform Homage (page 45). As you do the exercise, be aware of the way your energy centres open as you uncurl after the first movement and close again as you move down for the second one.

Meditation
On page 79 we moved from the root centre to the pelvic centre, discovering that there is a change in the level of awareness – physical at the root centre, and emotional at the pelvic centre.

Begin again at the pelvic centre and follow the energy upwards to your navel centre and then your heart centre. Use your hands, if you like. All these centres have an emotional ambience, as you would expect, but you may find it difficult to move away from your heart centre. There is a block here too, known in the tradition as the preserver's block (*vishnu granthi*). That is because the ambience beyond your heart

centre is mental. We shall return to this on page 83, but for now move back down through today's centres so that they can close.

Relaxation
Lie face down and imagine that you can feel the sun's rays on your shoulder blades. This time, feel them down to your waist and to the base of your spine.

Benefits
Homage is probably the most intense way to feel energy moving as you move. It's something you could do whenever you feel you need an astral boost.

Anyone can reach perfection in yoga,
regardless of age or health,
but only with determination.

Hathayoga Pradipika 1:64

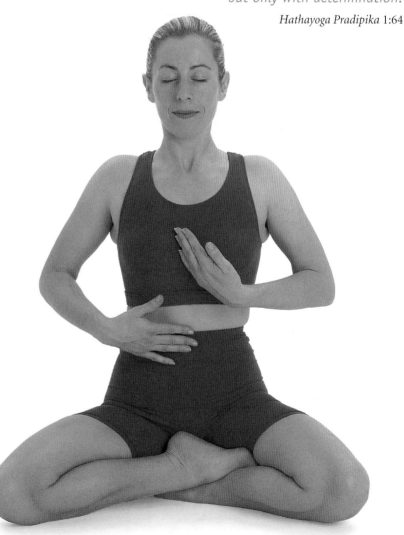

49 The Cobra

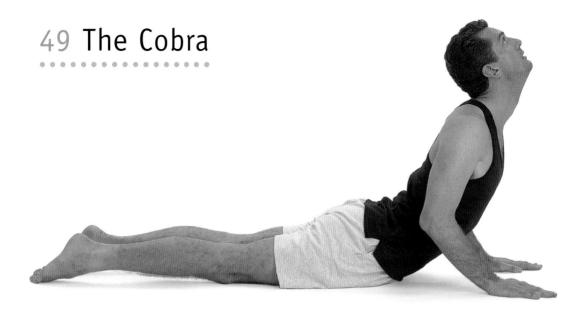

Becoming Aware

Lie face down and feel really relaxed on your mat. Total harmlessness (page 80) has an even more far-reaching, positive side: the idea that we need to have an approach to ourselves and our world that is totally devoid of harm so that we act as if we had never learned what harm is. In Yoga it's believed that we can actually go back to our primal innocence, and perhaps that is what you are beginning to do in your meditations.

Limbering

Perform Limber 9 (page 13).

Posture

Today's posture is the Cobra (*bhujangasana*). Assume the Prone Corpse (page 19) and bring your legs together with your hands under your shoulders. As you inhale, lift your eyes, then your head and then your chest upwards until your navel is just touching the floor and you are looking straight up to the ceiling. Exhale and let your chest move forwards a little and your arms bend slightly at the elbow.

After a pause, come down again, exhaling and turning your forehead down to the floor (to ease your neck).

Do not straighten your arms in this pose – you are meant to be lifting from the base of your spine, not pushing up with your hands. It's a demanding pose, but rewarding for your back, legs, chest and your shoulders. This is an excellent pose for opening your heart centre and your throat centre.

After a rest in the Prone Corpse, perform the Cobra twice more.

After you have performed this pose you need to move your body in the opposite direction and rest there for about 12 seconds.

Relaxation

Relax in the Prone Corpse position.

✳ Adaptations

A good alternative is the Sphynx. The difference is that you lay your forearms on the mat and only come up a little way, looking straight ahead.

• Precautions

If you have neck problems, keep your head facing forwards or try the Adaptation.

50 A Giant Leap

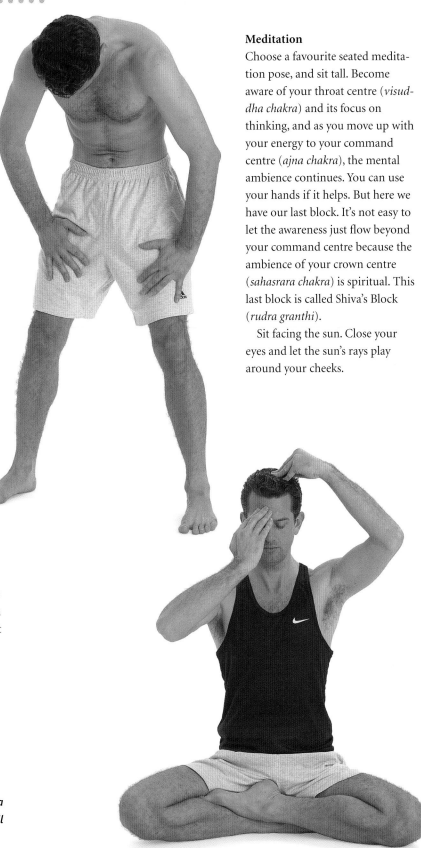

Becoming Aware

Walk into your space but remain standing. Pause to collect your thoughts and move into the Mountain.

The Giant Leap

To open the energy channels in your abdomen perform the first version of the Giant Leap (*uddiyana dhauti*). Move to an astride position and slightly bend your knees – you can turn your feet out a bit if you like. Put your palms flat on your upper thighs. Inhale. As you exhale, bend forwards, taking support from your hands, and look at your navel.

Inhale. As you exhale, pull your navel strongly back to your spine and up under your ribs. Stay in position, with your lungs empty, for a few seconds. Don't breathe in yet but release your abdomen. Breathe in and stand up. Stay astride for another round.

You will feel how strongly this opens up the energy channels in your abdomen.

Breathing

Notice how the Giant Leap affects the Bee Breath (page 75). Perform it gently but efficiently, for the last time. You can include it your personal choice later.

Directing Inner Energy

Perform the Space-walker (page 47) to energize your sinuses.

• Precautions

If you are pregnant or have a hernia or high blood pressure, Shining Skull (page 41) is a good alternative.

Meditation

Choose a favourite seated meditation pose, and sit tall. Become aware of your throat centre (*visuddha chakra*) and its focus on thinking, and as you move up with your energy to your command centre (*ajna chakra*), the mental ambience continues. You can use your hands if it helps. But here we have our last block. It's not easy to let the awareness just flow beyond your command centre because the ambience of your crown centre (*sahasrara chakra*) is spiritual. This last block is called Shiva's Block (*rudra granthi*).

Sit facing the sun. Close your eyes and let the sun's rays play around your cheeks.

51 More Dancing

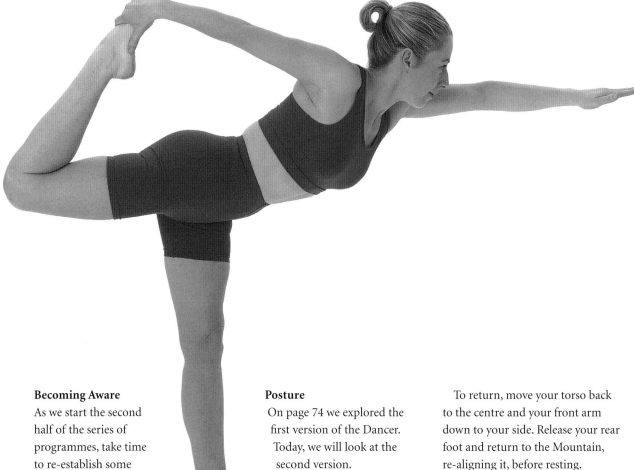

Becoming Aware

As we start the second half of the series of programmes, take time to re-establish some basic principles.

Begin this programme by walking elegantly to the centre of your space and standing quietly. Make the Gesture of Greeting if you like. Listen to your breathing and send out some good thoughts to your family and friends.

Consider the second of the yogic moral values, truth (*satya*). Yoga is always positive about things. Yogic truth means being objective and not feeling vulnerable but seeing people and things as they really are, and not feeling threatened or anxious about them.

Limbering

Perform Limber 1 (page 9).

Posture

On page 74 we explored the first version of the Dancer. Today, we will look at the second version.

Assume the Mountain (page 14), paying particular attention to being properly balanced. If necessary, use a chairback to help you balance. Lift your right knee, lightly grasp the ankle with your right hand and take it under you to the rear, moving it in close to your right buttock.

Raise your left arm to shoulder height, and incline your torso forwards, following your left hand out in front of you and lifting your rear arm and foot, to keep you balanced.

Your pose is complete when your forward arm and rear arm are in line. Stay in pose, breathing quietly, while the benefits work, and you feel as graceful as you look.

To return, move your torso back to the centre and your front arm down to your side. Release your rear foot and return to the Mountain, re-aligning it, before resting.

If balancing is a real problem, perform the two parts separately, but whatever you decide, perform the pose again now, with the confidence that you know what to do and have done it once.

Relaxation

After all that standing, lie down on your back with your knees raised for an extra-deep relaxation.

> **• Precautions**
>
> *Don't persist with balances if you are unsteady – you will only become anxious and unsteadier. Do the poses bit by bit – legs first, on their own, and then arms on their own.*

52 The Sound of Peace

Becoming Aware
Walk elegantly to the centre of your space or mat, where your energy imprint is now firmly established, and assume a classical seated pose or just kneel.

Opening Energy Channels
Perform Alternate Nostril Breathing (page 35).

Breathing
Today we are going to learn a new technique, Piercing the Moon (*chandra bedha*), which we will gradually build up over the next five programmes. Sit tall, and lay the middle finger of your right hand on the right side of your nose, and then breathe in through the left nostril. Now lay that finger on the left side of your nose and breathe out through the right side. Repeat the exercise.

Left and right are essential ideas in yoga. Left represents the moon, coolness, feminine and Shakti; right represents the Sun, warmth, masculine, and Shiva. You also have a left astral channel (*ida nadi*, the cool channel), and a right astral channel (*pingala nadi*, the sun-tanned channel).

Directing Inner Energy
Perform the Seal of the Container (page 49).

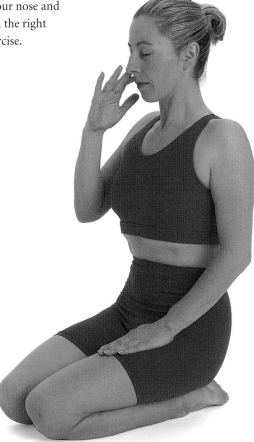

Meditation
The yoga word for peace is *shanti*. Say *shanti* to yourself, several times. Get used to the idea and then say it out loud. People who practise yoga believe that saying words such as this is good for you because it underlines the meaning, it stimulates the throat centre (*visuddha chakra*), and the vibrations work in your body. Doing this is called *mantra* (a repeated sound that carries a meaning).

Relaxation
Imagine your are taking a relaxing walk with a few friends and come upon a little cottage, with the door standing ajar and people coming out, obviously happy. Pass them and smile as you go in, and find yourself in a room with red walls, red curtains, a red carpet ... everything is red ... and as you stand looking, it's almost as if there's a red glow over everything, including you and your friends. The glow seems to make you feel strong, balanced and firm – and you remember that red is the colour of your root centre (*muladhara chakra*).

53 The Cow's Head

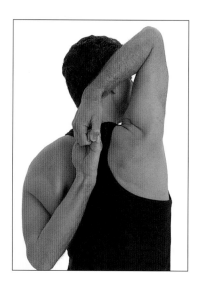

Becoming Aware
Traditional yoga teaching holds that in meditation we become aware of the inner essence of the object of our contemplation. When we meditate on a candle, we begin by concentrating on it, observing its every feature, but as we move into contemplation and stop using our brains, we can 'look inside' the candle and discover its essence.

Limbering
Perform Limber 2 (page 10).

Posture
You will need a scarf or sock for today's posture, which is known as the Cow's Head or Cow's Face (*gomukhasana*). Begin by assuming the Rock (page 16). Can you cross your knees? Can you put one knee (it doesn't matter which) over the other and sit between your feet? If you can, move your feet out slightly to each side, they will begin to look like the cow's horns. If you cannot, stay in the Rock, and let the cow do without horns. If you have managed it, see which knee is on top.

Take a scarf or sock in your other hand (the opposite hand to the knee on top, see photograph below) and move that arm up in front of you and over behind you, so that the scarf hangs down your back. Take your other arm out to the side and round behind you. Grasp the scarf or sock with your fingers.

If you don't need the scarf, let it drop to the mat and intertwine your fingers instead (see close-up photograph right).

Inhale deeply and look at your raised arm. Exhale to the front. Repeat that. Don't let your head rotate or bend forwards. Now you have completed one round and should do it all again on the other side. When you have finished, be careful how you separate your knees – they may be tired or stiff.

Relaxation
The easiest pose for relaxation from where you are is the Child (page 66).

> **• Precautions**
>
> *Proceed carefully with this pose if you have painful shoulders. It isn't compulsory to link your fingers.*

> **✳ Adaptations**
>
> *If your knees are stiff stay in the Rock.*

54 Peace Chant

Becoming Aware
Move elegantly to your space or mat and sit tall in the centre.

Opening Energy Channels
Perform Candle Gazing (page 37).

Breathing
Today we are going to look at Piercing the Moon (page 85) again, especially the counting sequence. Sit tall and breathe fully out. Inhale through your left nostril for 6, hold for 14, breathe out through your right nostril for 8, and wait for 4. Do that again several times, until the process becomes familiar. Make sure that the breaths last for the whole time you have allowed for them and use all three parts of your body. The inhalation should be abdomen 2, ribcage 2, upper chest 2; keep all three areas open and full for 14. The exhalation should be chest 2, ribcage 2, abdomen 4; keep all three areas closed and empty for 4.

Directing Inner Energy
Today's *mudra* is Looking at the Void (page 51).

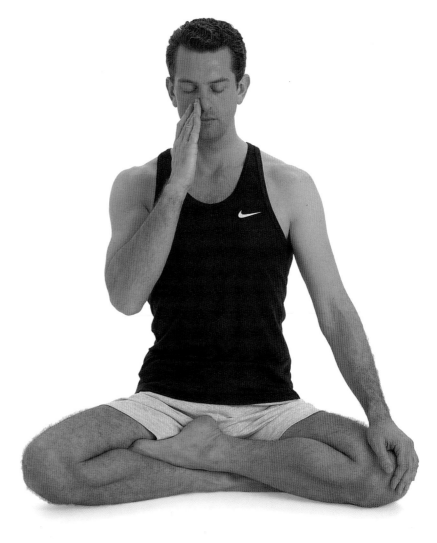

Meditation
Change your pose if you wish. Inhale and start saying *shanti* over and over again. Let your ordinary speaking voice become more dramatic. Imagine that you want to be heard in the next street, and start declaiming *shanti, shanti, shanti*. It's only a short step from declaiming to chanting. Sing the word now – it doesn't matter what note it is or even if it actually sounds like a note or not. Just utter the word *ssshhhaaannntttiii* ... and then go on, only stopping for breath.

Don't stop suddenly. Quieten down and rest in silence for a few moments. Chanting stimulates every part of you, especially your astral centres, so give them time to calm down and close down. We close astral centres when we are not doing yoga practice because they are rather special, and we should open them only on special occasions and because it's not a good idea for them to be open when we are busy doing other things and cannot give them our full attention.

Relaxation
Imagine that you are visiting the cottage again. Walk through the red room and through a door leading into an orange room. Marvel at the effect of the orange furnishings, the orange carpet and the orange glow that lies over everything, including you and your friends. Begin to feel awake and emotionally excited. Remember that orange is the colour of your pelvic centre. Let the colour fade before you conclude your practice, otherwise your pelvic centre will not close.

55 Turning to the West

Becoming Aware

Sit in the centre of your mat and lean back. Open your chest with a deep inhalation and tuck your abdomen well in on the exhalation. Stay like that for 12 seconds, or as long as you can.

Think about the third yogic moral value, honesty (*asteya*). This is about not deceiving other people and not deceiving yourself. It's also about living in the real world. As far as yoga is concerned, it means being honest about how supple you are and whether, for instance, you should be doing such dynamic breathing with your hernia. You will make the best progress if you use the right techniques for your own circumstances.

Limbering

Perform Limber 3 (page 10).

Posture

On page 78 we looked at the Seated Forward Bend, which is also known as Extending your Western Side. Today we will explore the Rotated Seat Forward Bend or Turning your Western Side Around

(*parivritta paschimottanasana*). If you had difficulty with the earlier posture, look at the alternative suggested on page 78 and do not try this pose.

Begin by assuming the Pole (page 17). Inhale deeply, raising your arms above your head. As you exhale, bring your spine forwards, folding at your hips, and keeping your back flat. Rest when you have moved down as far as is comfortable for you. After another inhalation, see if you can move a little further and curl your middle fingers around your big toes.

Now comes the turning part. Breathing quietly, change your arms over, so that your hands are holding the opposite big toes. Look to see which arm is on the top. Lift this arm and make a space under it. Turn your head to that side and look through the space. This will work only if you turn your torso and shoulders as well, so that your upper shoulder is well up and over your head and your lower arm is

near the space between your legs. This is quite demanding, and it is important that you don't expect too much success until you can perform the standard version.

To conclude the pose, return to the standard forward position, and rest in that, before uncurling and returning to the Pole.

Relaxation

Resting today is probably best done lying prone to balance all the work you have done with your spine. You could also usefully lie supine and cuddle your knees to ease your back.

● **Precautions**

Be honest with yourself about your ability to do forward extensions.

✱ **Adaptations**

The version with raised knees (see page 78) is an excellent alternative to this posture and is good as a forward extension.

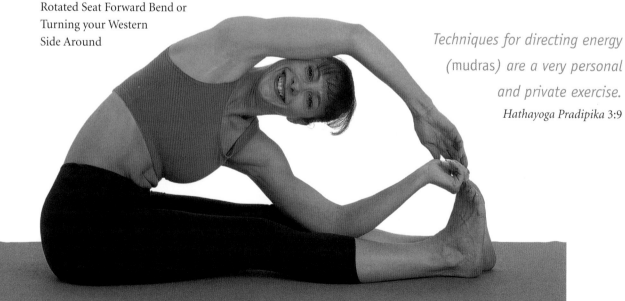

Techniques for directing energy (mudras) are a very personal and private exercise.

Hathayoga Pradipika 3:9

56 The Sound of the Universe

Becoming Aware
Settle calmly and perhaps make the Gesture of Greeting.

Opening Inner Channels
Open the astral channels with Head-furrow Cleansing (page 39).

Breathing
Today we will proceed with Piercing the Moon, but add the muscular locks (*bandhas*) which are just like those in Piercing the Sun (pages 65 and 67). Breathing quietly, tighten your pelvic muscles to make the Root Lock (page 35) and release it. Inhaling, turn your head down, from the top of your neck, to make the Waterpipe Lock (page 37), and release it. Exhaling, tuck your abdomen back against your spine and up under your ribs to make the Lock that Flies Up (page 39). Release it.

Now let's put it all together. Inhale for 6 through your left nostril. Apply the Root Lock (take 2). Apply the Waterpipe Lock (take 2). Wait with the lungs full for 12 more. Release the Waterpipe Lock (take 2). Release the Root Lock (take 2). Exhale through the right nostril with the Lock that Flies Up for 8 seconds. Put your right hand back on your thigh (take 2). Release the lock (take 2). And rest.

Directing Inner Energy
Today perform the Seal of Shiva (page 53).

Meditation
You've had some practice in chanting, so now here's the best known chant (*mantra*) in the tradition. Inhale and then make the sound *aaaahh*; it will feel as if it's coming from your abdomen. Now make the sound *uuuuuuugh*; it will feel as if it's coming from your chest. Finally, make the sound *mmmmm-mmmmm* with closed lips; it will feel as if it's coming from your head.

Now make all three sounds in one breath. Inhale fully first, then chant *aaaaaaa-uuuuuuu-mmmm-mmm*. You have chanted *aum* (or *om*), the sound of the Universe.

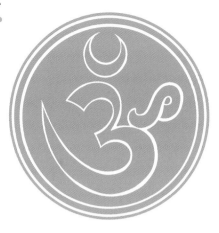

The 'Om' symbol

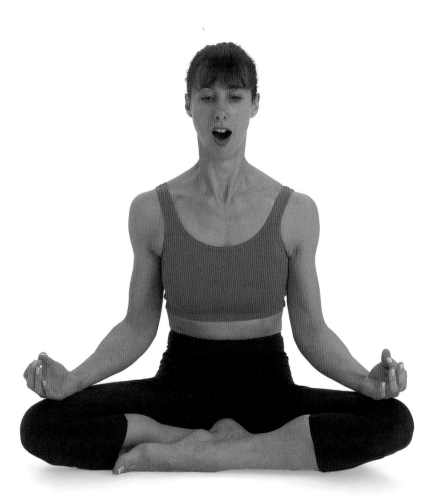

Relaxation
Imagine that you are visiting the cottage again. This time go to the yellow room. Stand in the yellow glow and start to feel receptive to emotion and not afraid of it. You feel as if you want to feel more and more emotion and to express it. Yellow is, of course, the colour of your navel astral centre (*manipura chakra*), the centre of feeling.

57 Gone with the Wind

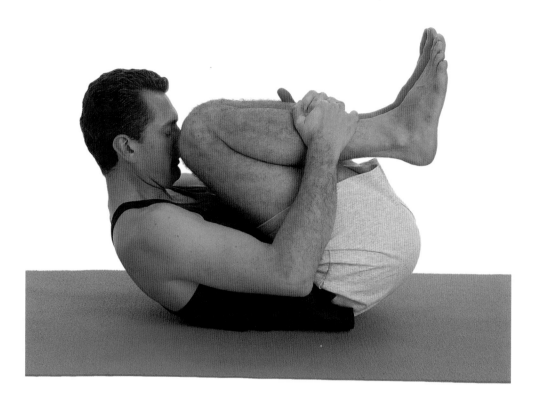

Becoming Aware

Settle into your quiet yoga mood and think further about yogic honesty (*asteya*). It is also about who is doing the yoga. In these programmes it is you on your own – it's your time and place, and it's your progress and yours alone that should concern you. This is not the time to make comparisons with other people you know who do yoga, and remember that the photographs here are offered only as information and encouragement.

Limbering

Perform Limber 8 (page 12).

Posture

Today's pose, the Wind Pose (*vatnyasana*), was used originally to aid digestion, but it has become a great favourite for easing out the spine and massaging the abdomen. Begin by assuming the Corpse (page 18). Inhale. As you exhale, bring your left knee up to your chest, without holding it – see how far it will come by itself. Breathe quietly as you lay your left hand on your shin and your right hand on your foot. See if you can touch your chest with your knee and your buttock with your heel.

Inhale again. As you exhale, bring your nose to your knee. It may actually touch your knee, but it's getting the nose near the knee that really matters. Stay in the pose to let the energy work and the benefits happen.

Lay your head down again, inhaling, and then, breathing quietly, release your hands but leave the knee where it is for a moment, before gently laying it down again on the mat and resting. Do all this again, on the other side.

Repeat the movements, but with both legs. Put one hand on each shin and see if you can make contact between your knees and your chest or between your heels and your buttocks, or both. Bring your nose to the divide between your knees (or just inside it). That's one round. Do two or three rounds if you have time.

After you have performed this pose you need to move your body in the opposite direction and rest in the new position for about 12 seconds.

Relaxation

Rest in the Corpse.

58 More Universal Sound

Becoming Aware
Assume the Pole (page 17) and quietly reflect on your programme for today.

Opening Energy Channels
Remain in the Pole and perform the Cleansing with Internal Fire (page 43).

Breathing
With your astral energy channels now wide open, perform Piercing the Moon (page 85), not worrying too much about the count but giving a lot of attention to the locks (page 89). Once energy has begun to move, you can direct it where you want it by performing the locks with an awareness of their nature and function: the Root Lock (page 35) energizes your pelvic area; the Waterpipe Lock (page 37) energizes your upper torso; and the Lock that Flies Up (page 39) energizes your abdomen.

Directing Inner Energy
Hear all the inner sounds of astral energy by performing the Seal of the Six Openings (page 55).

Meditation
Inhale deeply, then chant *aaaaa-uuuuummmmm*. Become aware of what *aum* (*om*) really is. It is the name of the universal godhead in the ancient yogic tradition, and in a way, you are invoking your god when you chant it. Don't worry if you're not sure about that, because it's also reckoned to be just the sound the universe makes, so you are just tuning in to the universe.

Inhale deeply and chant *om* again, making it what you want it to be.

Relaxation
Imagine you are in the green room in the cottage and feel your heart leap. Green is the colour of your astral heart centre (*anahata chakra*). Meditating on the colour and knowing its connection with the *chakra* will be enough to open up the centre.

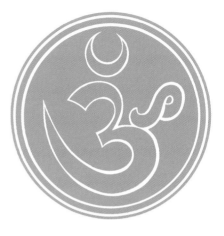

The 'Om' symbol

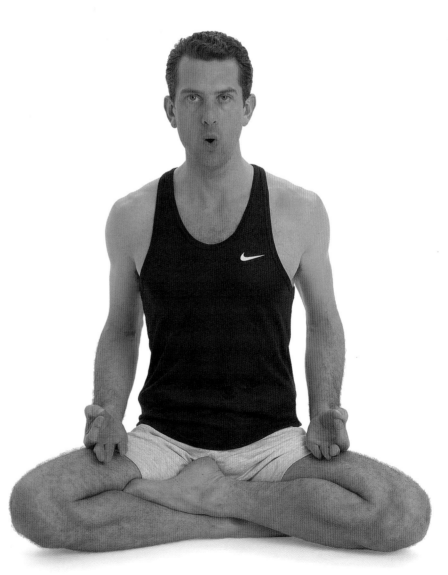

59 The Locust

Becoming Aware

Settle on your mat in the Prone Corpse pose and notice that a great deal of today's programme is about lifting tops and tails. The next yogic moral value is self-discipline (*brahmacharya*). The word, which actually means 'disciple of god', implies that in order to succeed in yoga you must take your cue from god's disciples and sort out your priorities.

Limbering

Perform Limber 9 (page 13).

Posture

Begin today's posture, the Locust (*salabhasana*), by assuming the Prone Corpse (page 19).

Take your arms to your sides and put your legs together. Inhale. As you exhale, lift your left leg from the mat, keeping it straight if you can. To achieve the full lift you will find that your left hip lifts up as well. That's all right but make sure your body doesn't rotate over to the right. Don't breathe in yet. Lower the leg to the mat, breathe in and rest. Try not to press down with your arms but make your lower back muscles and buttocks do the work. Now do it all again on the other side.

These are just steps to the full pose, so now do it all once more, but with both legs. Remember not to use your arms and remember to exhale as you lift your legs up and

Benefits
As well as the benefit of lifting, while you are basically at rest, you will find that the pose massages your abdomen.

not to breathe in again until your legs are back on the mat. Return to the Corpse for a short rest.

After you have performed this pose you need to move your body in the opposite direction and rest in the new position for about 12 seconds.

Relaxation

Lie for a few moments on your front and let all your muscles go soft.

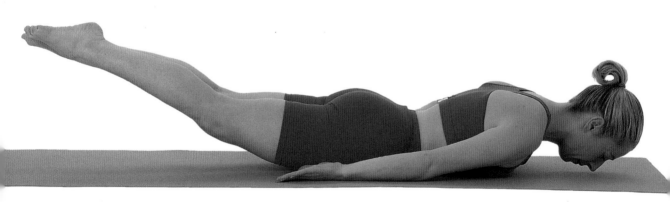

• Precautions

Don't be tempted to push yourself up into the Locust with your hands. It's sometimes done this way, but it's really a different pose and doesn't use the lower spine in the same way.

If you have a weak back do not attempt to lift both legs at once.

If you are pregnant you should avoid prone poses.

✳ Adaptations

More Rolling Around (page 62) is a good alternative programme.

60 The Blue Room

Becoming Aware
Assume the Mountain and feel strong as well as relaxed.

Opening Energy Channels
Open your astral channels with the Giant Leap (page 83).

Breathing
Adopt a seated meditation pose for your last time with Piercing the Moon. It doesn't matter if you don't quite get the details exactly right (see page 85 to refresh your memory), but do think about the breath entering your left nostril (the moon, cool, feminine).

Directing Inner Energy
Fix the energy where you want it with the Great Seal (page 57).

Meditation
Chant *om* to your heart's content, but today, be aware that in yogic tradition, the three letters of *om* – *a-u-m* – have their own individual attributes and together, when they form a complete word, they have some extra attributes:
A represents fire, the earth, the past and intuition;
U represents wind, the atmosphere, the present and intellect;
M represents the sun, the sky, the future and thoughts;
AUM is the godhead within you, the very first word and the 'forever' thought.

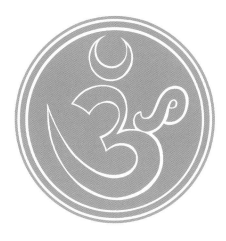

The 'Om' symbol

Relaxation
Imagine you are in the blue room, feel that you want to express yourself, to speak and listen, to make contact and be contacted – all the attributes of your astral throat centre (*visuddha chakra*).

A is for the waking state
U is for the dream state
M is for dreamless sleep
but AUM is for 'Yoga Nidra'
the bliss of non-awareness.
Mandukya Upanishad 9:12

61 The Triangle

Becoming Aware
Walk onto your mat and thought-fully assume the Mountain (page 15).

Limbering
Perform Limber 1 (page 9).

Posture
Today's posture is another classic pose, the Forward-facing Triangle (*utthita trikonasana*). It extends one side of your body and compresses the other. It's vital that you do not rotate your torso as you perform.

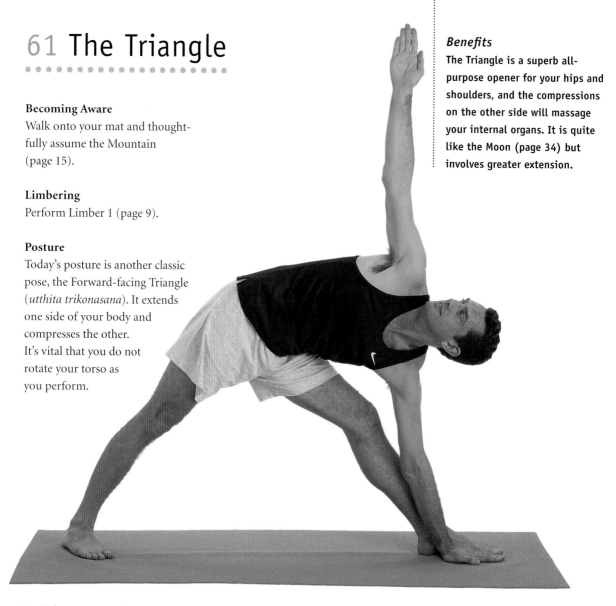

Benefits
The Triangle is a superb all-purpose opener for your hips and shoulders, and the compressions on the other side will massage your internal organs. It is quite like the Moon (page 34) but involves greater extension.

Begin by assuming the Mountain (page 15). Step out, one leg at a time, to a really wide stride, but remain standing tall. We will go to the left first, so turn out your left foot on its heel and your right foot on its toes. If your hips and shoulders turned to the left as you did that, turn fully back to the front. You should already be feeling a good stretch on the muscles inside your left thigh. Check that you are still standing tall. Inhale and raise both your arms to shoulder height.

As you exhale, move your torso to your left but don't rotate. When you have moved fully to your left,

turn your torso downwards, so that you can lay your left palm either on the mat by your left foot or on your left ankle or on your left shin. Your right arm will be above your head. Breathe quietly and check that you are properly supported by your left foot and left hand. Check that your right arm is directly above you and that your right hip and right shoulder are fully open.

Stay in pose, breathing quietly and looking straight ahead. If balancing is hard, lean back a little on your right foot.

To come back, continue breathing quietly and raise your torso back up to the centre. Lower your

arms, and resume a good tall Mountain pose.

Repeat the entire exercise on the other side. And that is one round. Perform another round.

Relaxation
Relax in the Corpse.

• Precautions

If your back is weak, be careful how you perform the Triangle.

* Adaptations

The Moon (page 34) is a good alternative.

94

62 Working with Beads

Becoming Aware

Choose a seated pose but extend your repertoire and make yourself more supple by deciding on a pose in which you are not yet completely comfortable.

For example, if you can happily sit in the Easy Pose on two blocks, you could try sitting in the same way but on one block or you could sit on two blocks, but in the Pose of the Expert. Then go on to the Half Lotus and finally, to the Full Lotus with no blocks.

Opening Energy Channels

Perform Alternate Nostril Breathing (page 35) to open your energy channels.

Breathing

We reach a special way of breathing today – still breathing or the Silence of the Solitary Breath (*kevala kumbhaka*). Most of the yogic breathing that we do is strictly controlled and is known as structured breathing (*sahita kumbhaka*). Still breathing is when the breathing is so still and silent, it's almost as if it had stopped altogether. The problem with it is that as soon as you notice that your breathing is still, you feel that you must start breathing deeply. It's a good test of the level of your awareness, and it happens best when you aren't aware of it at all. See if you can let your breathing slow down and become truly soft and shallow. We will look at this again on page 96.

Directing Inner Energy

Today, try the Big Poker (page 59) in the Easy Pose or the Pose of the Expert.

Meditation

You will need a string of beads for today's programme. Take the beads and move them through the fingers of your right hand. Can you make them move at about one a second? As you pass them through, say *shanti* once per bead. This is known as 'chanting a repeated *mantra* with beads' (*mantra japa mala*). If the beads are strung in a circle, run easily through your fingers and there are 54 or 108 of them, then you are fully equipped to use this programme, which we will look at again on page 97.

The magic happens when you are still.
Traditional Yogic teaching

Benefits
Silent, still breathing can be relaxing, especially if you aren't disturbed when it starts to get dynamic. Asthmatics can benefit hugely from still breathing.

Relaxation

Imagine you are in a room decked out in indigo, the intense colour of your command centre (*ajna chakra*) in your forehead. Begin to feel yourself thinking clearly and decisively, but don't forget to see the indigo colour fade from sight so that the astral command centre closes down.

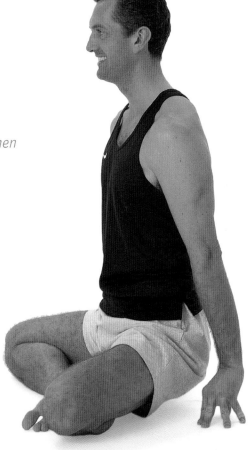

63 The Dove

Becoming Aware
Become quiet today in the Rock (page 16). The last of the yogic moral values is the idea of not being greedy (*aparigraha*). Of course, this has the obvious meaning of being satisfied with what you've got and not taking more than your fair share, but there is also an inner, more personal meaning – that being greedy suggests there may be a hurt of some kind below the surface and that greed arises out of anxiety.

Limbering
Perform Limber 2 (page 10).

Posture
Today's pose is the Dove. The name derives from its shape and its graceful elegance, and it has a number of important steps, making it an excellent posture for physical discipline.

Begin by assuming the Rock (page 16). Breathing quietly, lean forwards and place your hands on the mat. Slide your right leg back so that it is extended behind you and you are kneeling on your left heel.

Place your hands, one on the other, on top of your left thigh and support your spine as you kneel, tall and vertical. You will feel the effects of this on your lower back, so listen to your body and don't do too much.

Finally, still breathing quietly, place your right hand on your right calf, way out behind you, and walk the fingers along, perhaps on an exhalation. Turn to look at that hand. Hold your pose, pause and be still, perhaps with still breathing (page 95).

Do it all again on the other side. That is one round. If you have time, perform one or two more rounds.

Relaxation
Try resting in the Child (page 66), mostly because it's so handy after all that kneeling.

● **Precautions**

Weak knees will not like this programme at all.

✱ **Adaptations**

A good alternative would be the Cobra (page 82) or the Locust (page 92).

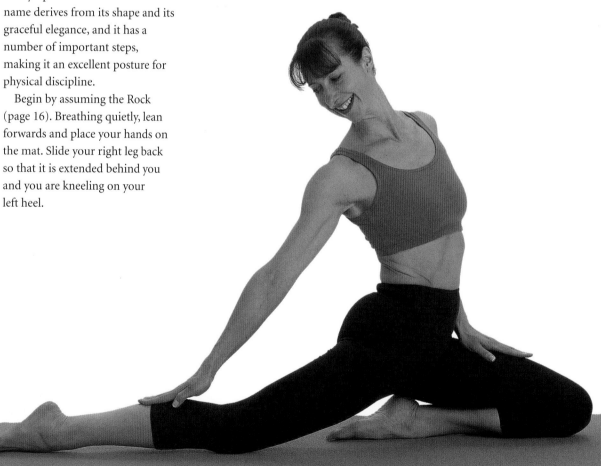

96

64 Crown of Violets

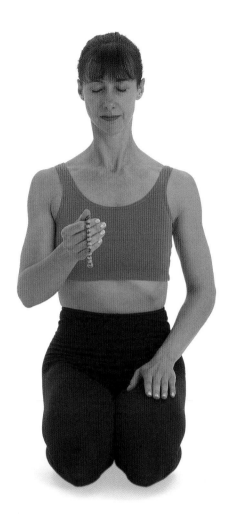

Becoming Aware
Perform the Pose of the Expert on one block as your calm opening pose today.

Opening Energy Channels
Clear the way for astral energy, especially in your sinuses, by performing Candle Gazing (page 37).

Breathing
Today we will continue to look at still breathing (page 95), which is believed to be the only effective accompaniment to meditation.

Inhale deeply and watch your breath gradually settle. Exhale deeply and watch your breath recover and settle. Finally, see if the breath will just subside by itself, even with your attention on it.

The time you are spending on your breath is a little meditation, which is one of the most ancient of all meditations.

Directing Inner Energy
Prepare to perform the Seal of the Dawn Horse (page 61). As you ride along – try for 12 bounces at a time, with rests between – be aware of each downward movement as a boost for the energy in your lowest astral centres, the root centre (*muladhara chakra*) and the pelvic centre (*svadisthana chakra*).

• Precautions
Do not perform the Seal of the Dawn Horse if you have weak knees or a bad back.

✴ Adaptations
The Big Poker (page 59) is a good alternative.

Meditation
Take your beads again and hold them in your right hand. It would be good if one bead was larger than the rest or if there were some way of knowing when you have

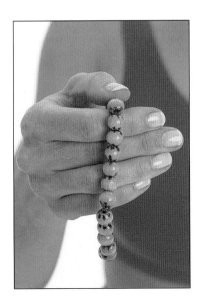

been right round the circle. Move the beads through your fingers, towards you, one bead at a time, at intervals of a bead a second if you can. As the beads move, quietly say *shanti* on each bead. The effect of chanting a repeated *mantra* with beads is that you will probably begin by concentrating (*dharana*), but as you continue, this will subtly change to a more gentle and general awareness (*dhyana*). This is a classical meditation method.

Relaxation
Imagine that you have finally arrived in a room richly decked out in hues of violet. You feel excited, but in a strange way – you are totally fulfilled. Violet is the colour of your crown centre (*sahasrara chakra*). Remember to see the violet fade as the crown centre closes.

65 Head to Knee

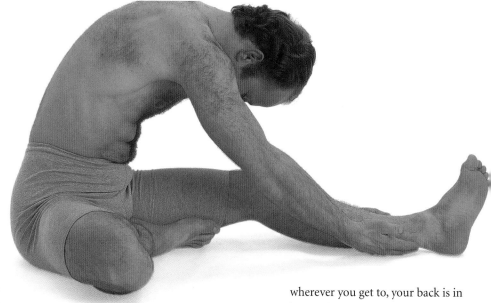

Becoming Aware

Assume an informal version of the Pole (page 17), lean slightly back and breathe deeply but slowly into your abdomen. This is a good way to 'slow down', physically and emotionally, ready for your practice. Think again about the last of the yogic moral values, the state of not being greedy. The traditional view is that if you pay full attention to your techniques as you practice, you will feel fulfilled and contented – which is the positive side of this state. It is not so much about making an effort not to be greedy, as being so happily occupied that you forget to be greedy.

Limbering

Perform Limber 3 (page 10).

Posture

Today's pose is the Head to Knee Pose (*janu sirsasana*), which is another major classical pose that rewards careful performance. Being by assuming the Pole (page 17). Using only your right hand (keep your left hand in Pole position, to keep you sitting tall), bring your right foot close in to your groin. Don't reach forwards to collect it – bend it as far as your can and then use your hand. Stay in a tall Pole pose. When your foot is in position, lay your left knee down on the floor. If your thigh muscles won't let your knee go all the way down, try turning your torso a little way towards your left side. If you still have problems, try carefully turning your left leg over so that it lies on its inner side.

The rest of the pose is sometimes performed rather like the Seated Forward Bend (page 78), but today we will really aim to put our heads on our knees. Turn your torso, so that you are facing your outstretched leg. Inhale. As you exhale, curl your back down so that your head moves down towards your knee. Let your hands rest lightly, palms up, on the floor on each side of your leg.

Before you attempt to touch your kneecap with your nose, make sure that both your elbows are on the mat. This will ensure that your back is correctly in line. It doesn't matter if you can't go far down, but it's really important that wherever you get to, your back is in line with your leg, and your shoulders are level.

Pause in the pose with still breathing (page 95). After a few moments (say 12 seconds), inhale and gently see if your back and thigh muscles will let you down any further. Pause again. This is the static, meditational part of the pose, where you just let it do all its good things to you. When you are ready, slowly unwind yourself back to the Pole.

You will find that your sitting bones have moved, so lift yourself up and let them settle. Resume a tall Pole, before doing the entire exercise again on the other side and probably finding that you are not entirely symmetrical. That's one round. Perform another round with both sides.

Relaxation

Rest in the Corpse.

• Precautions

Do not be too dynamic when you perform this pose – you could easily hurt yourself.

66 Floating in Warm Currents

Becoming Aware
Sit in the Pose of the Expert with your hands in the Gesture of Wisdom. This pose will bring you calmness.

Opening Energy Channels
Perform Head-furrow Cleansing (page 39).

Breathing
Still sitting in the Pose of the Expert, allow still breathing to move you gently to and fro.

Directing Inner Energy
Change to the Rock if you are getting uncomfortable, then perform Homage (page 45), especially dwelling on the sensation at the base of your spine, where your root centre (*muladhara chakra*) resides.

Meditation
Change your pose again if you need to, adopting one that you can stay in for a few minutes without distraction. Concentrate (*dharana*) on your root *chakra*. Feel its physical position on your body. Recall its traditional name – *muladhara chakra* – and say it in your mind. Become aware of its function as the foundation of your being. Imagine that you are seated on a red velvet cushion. Let all these thoughts gently occupy your awareness and do not feel the need to form any more thoughts about it.

Benefits
Today's meditation is in the true classical style. We hope you enjoy it. You are now able to slip easily into meditation – and you can recall the experience whenever you wish, perhaps in moments of stress.

Sit for a few moments. Let time stop and give yourself a chance to have a glimpse of what it might be like to be in yogic bliss (*samadhi*).

Relaxation
After all that heady meditation, relax and imagine that you are floating on warm currents of scented water.

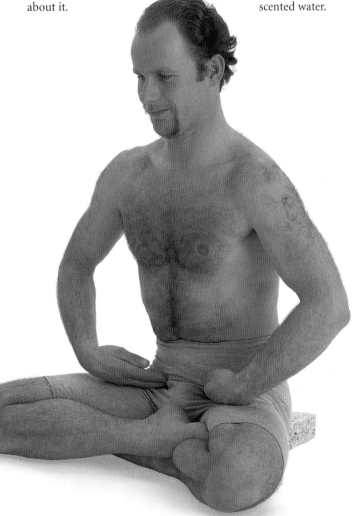

67 The Fish

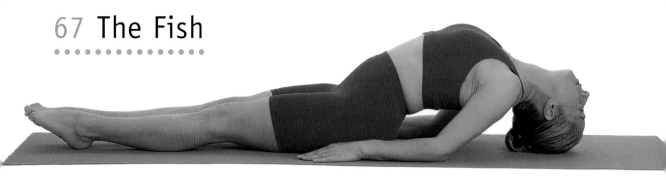

Becoming Aware

You can become calm in the Corpse but don't let yourself become sleepy. Think about the yogic moral values we have been exploring. The ancient teachers used to say that you should be able to prove that you had achieved them all before you start yoga studies. Nowadays, it's probably more realistic to say that you hope your yoga practice will help you to achieve some of them soon.

Limbering

Perform Limber 8 (page 12).

Posture

Today's pose is the Fish (*matsyasana*), and we will be looking at the simplest version. Assume the Corpse (page 18) and move to an alert Corpse pose, with your legs together and arms beside you, palms down. Gently breathe fully out. As you strongly inhale, arch your back and turn your head back to look behind you. Don't move your elbows out to support you, just let them bend slightly as you arch your back.

If you have a strong and supple neck, you will be able to rest on the crown of your head. Alternatively, let your head stay where it feels the most comfortable. Continue to breathe quietly.

To conclude the pose, move to the Corpse again by just lying down, bringing your spine down to the mat in stages, from the base to your neck. Notice how this opens your chest and your abdomen, stimulating your navel and heart centres.

After you have performed this pose you need to move your body in the opposite direction and rest in the new position for about 12 seconds.

• Precautions

Be very careful with your neck. Use the adaptation if you are unsure.

✴ Adaptations

A more secure way of using your arms to help you is to lift your left side a little from the mat, and slip your left arm right under your body, with your buttock or thigh resting on the back of your left hand. Repeat

this on the other side. Now you will find that you can lift your torso with more control and let your head down more safely. Slip your arms out when you have completed two rounds.

This pose can also be performed with your legs in any of the seated meditation poses.

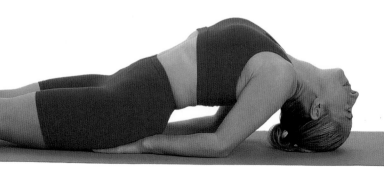

68 Using a Mandala

Becoming Aware

Sit in the Pose of the Expert with your hands in the Gesture of Wisdom.

Opening Energy Channels

Move slowly to a Mountain pose and perform the Giant Leap (page 83) to open the energy channels in your lower body. If you are able, perform two rounds.

Breathing

Move slowly back down into the Pose of the Expert with your hands in the Gesture of Wisdom. Hold this pose for about 2 minutes with the still breath, which should be beginning to be a habit with you by now.

Directing Inner Energy

To stimulate the energy in your sinuses, perform the Space-walker (page 47).

Meditation

When you were using a candle for meditation (page 45), you were taking your inspiration from an external object. You can also do this with flowers, a sunset or sunrise or a mandala (a design).

Here is a mandala of your root centre (*muladhara chakra*). Examine it closely, looking at all the details (*dharana*) and letting

your eyes rest on it, without thinking about it (*dhyana*). You may find that your eyes have closed at some point and that time has passed you by. This could be yogic bliss.

One of the ancient uses for mandalas was for visual education, as an alternative to talking or books. For a real devotee, every detail is deeply significant and you can practise bhakti yoga, the yoga of devotion, with a mandala.

Relaxation

Imagine you are floating on the warm currents of scented water.

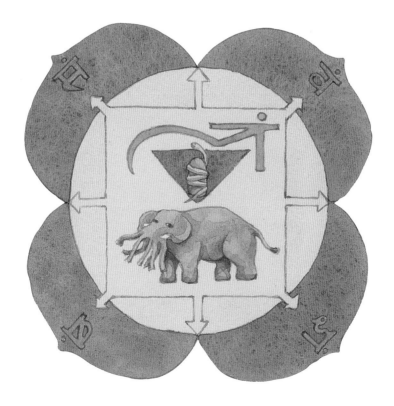

Muladhara Chakra:
the Base or Root Inner Energy Centre

69 The Golden Bow

Becoming Aware

Lie in the Prone Corpse. To accompany the yogic moral values, there is a set of yogic personal standards (*niyamas*). It was believed that you should be able to show evidence that you had mastered them all before attempting yoga studies. We will use them to show what yoga can do for you as you progress through the techniques.

Limbering

Perform Limber 9 (page 13).

Posture

Today's posture, the Bow (*dhanur-asana*), makes a good threesome with the Cobra (page 82) and the Locust (page 92). These lift the upper and lower parts of the body respectively; the Bow lifts both. Begin by assuming the Prone Corpse (page 19). Move to the alert form of the Prone Corpse with your legs together and your arms beside you, palms down. Lift your lower left leg and grasp it with your left hand. Do this with your other leg too. If you can't reach, loop a sock or a scarf around your foot to lift it into place. If necessary, keep this in place for the rest of the pose.

• Precautions

Do not attempt this pose if you are pregnant.

✷ Adaptations

If you need the sock or scarf, go on using it until you are more supple. It will mean that you can include the Bow in your practice without straining your spine. Alternatively, perform the Lucky Pose (page 50).

With your hands fitted securely around your feet, inhale. On the exhalation, draw your feet a little way back, until you feel your arms being extended and your shoulders beginning to lift. Don't pull too far – you have two more movements to make. Don't pull with your arms and don't bend your arms. Your legs are doing the work. Inhale again.

On the second exhalation, raise your feet towards the ceiling, but not too far. Feel the extension on your arms and the lift on your shoulders continuing to increase. Inhale again.

Benefits

The movements in this pose will tone and strengthen your whole body, and the rocking will massage and stimulate your internal organs.

On the last exhalation, lift your feet up and away from you to the rear. Feel the complete extension and lift. Maintain the pose. As you breathe, you will find that on the inhalations you will rock back a little, and on the exhalations you will rock forwards a little. Don't force the rocking movements – let your breathing do it.

To return to the Prone position, gently release your feet and lower your legs and shoulders. Don't be too strenuous – these are unfamiliar movements. Remember to balance after performing this pose.

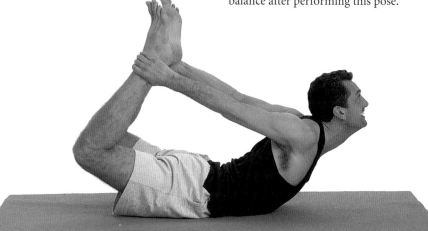

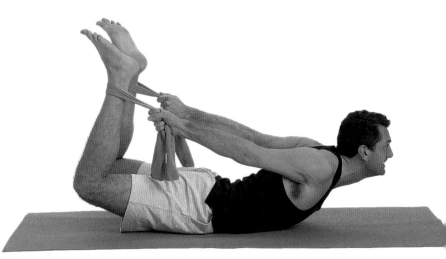

70 Twelve Giant Leaps

Becoming Aware
Try standing in the Mountain to become calm. Make the Gesture of Greeting to help.

Opening Energy Channels
To stimulate astral energy in your abdomen and help your digestion, perform the dynamic version of the Giant Leap. If you have a hiatus hernia, carefully perform the first version instead (page 83). For the dynamic version, step your legs out to a moderate width. On an exhalation, lean your torso forwards, supporting it by resting your palms on your thighs. Slowly but deeply inhale. As you exhale, look down at your abdomen and draw your navel back to your spine and up under your ribs. Stay in position with your lungs empty. Release your navel and draw it back again – a kind of flapping motion. Release your breath, come to a standing position and rest.

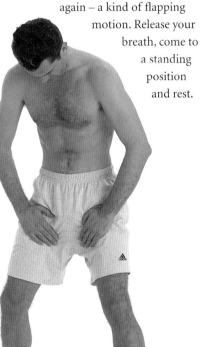

Inhale

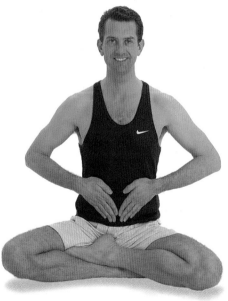

In the full technique, you need to do 12 of those flapping movements.

So, begin again and prepare to make your first flapping motion, but then go on to make 12 flaps. Release your breath, come to a standing position and rest.

You can always compromise with, say, six or three flaps, if 12 is too many for you. It's the repeated flaps that make this technique effective, stimulating your navel centre and toning your abdominal muscles and internal organs.

Exhale

Breathing
Settle into a favourite seated pose for your last look at still breathing (page 95).

Directing Inner Energy
Fix your astral energy with the Seal of the Container (page 49).

Meditation
Take your awareness to your pelvic centre. Feel its physical position on your body. Recall its traditional name – *svadisthana chakra* – and say it in your mind. Become aware of its function as the centre of your energy. Imagine that you have an orange silk sash around your hips. Now let yourself be content in the company of your root centre.

Relaxation
Imagine that you are going for a walk on your favourite beach. Listen to all the sounds of the sea, with the gulls and the waves ... listen but don't think!

71 The Reverse Triangle

Becoming Aware

Assume the Mountain and be still. The first of the five yogic personal standards is purity (*sauca*). In our modern terms, this means a kind of simplicity. It's about having an uncomplicated nature – a single-minded view of your life – and like all things in yoga, it's a positive quality.

Limbering

Perform Limber 1 (page 9).

Posture

To begin today's posture, the Reverse Triangle (*parivritta trikonasana*), assume the Mountain (page 15). Step out to a wide stride, using first one leg, then the other, so that you stay on the centre of your mat. Make the width at least as wide as is comfortable.

✳ Adaptations

If Triangles are not for you, perform the Fish (page 100) instead.

This move on its own will tone your thighs, and make you feel (and look) younger.

Stand tall, and turn your right foot out on its heel and your left foot out on its toes. Inhale and raise your arms to shoulder height. Exhale and check that you are facing fully to the front. Inhale again. On the exhalation, turn fully to your right so that you are facing your right leg.

Inhale, standing tall, and bend down towards your right foot, with your arms still at shoulder height and your back flat. When you have completed that movement, breathe quietly and place your left hand either on the mat by your right big toe or on the ankle or on the shin – or wherever it's comfortable. Look down to check that you are balanced and firm.

Benefits

This posture opens up the hips and shoulders and massages the waist and abdomen. The three lowest astral centres are also stimulated.

Turn to face behind you and raise your right arm up directly above your head. Carefully look up to check the position of your right arm. Complete the pose by looking directly behind you, neither up nor down. If you feel unsteady, press down on your rear foot. Stay in pose if you can, to allow time for the benefits to work.

To return, breathe quietly and return to the sideways flat back position, before lifting yourself up to the sideways-facing standing position. Turn back to the front, lower your arms and turn your feet to the front (by turning your left foot first, on its toes, and then your right foot, on its heel).

Rest for a few moments in this position, before preparing to perform the whole exercise again, on the other side. That was one round. If all went well, perform another round while the details are familiar.

Relaxation

Rest today in the Child (page 66).

72 Cooling Breath

Benefits
Perhaps the greatest benefit of any yoga practice is that you are engrossed in something simple for at least 10 minutes, and while your attention is occupied like this, your body, mind and emotions can rest and you feel deeply refreshed when it's over.

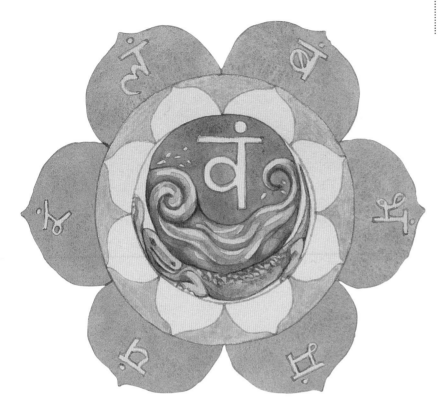

Svadisthana Chakra:
the Pelvic or Sacral Inner Energy Centre

Becoming Aware
Assume the Rock (page 16) for all today's techniques.

Opening Energy Channels
Stay in the Rock for Alternate Nostril Breathing (page 35).

Breathing
To stimulate cooling energies around your sinuses, perform the Cooling Breath again. Inhale gently. As you exhale, put out your tongue and curl up the tip, as if you were collecting raindrops.

Inhale through your mouth, with your tongue extended. Feel how cool that is. Hold your breath, with your lips together, and exhale through both nostrils.

Now do it again, with a count. Inhale gently for 4. Exhale for 4, extending your tongue. Inhale through your tongue for 8. Hold the breath fully for 8. Exhale through both nostrils for 8.

Directing Inner Energy
Perform today's *mudra*, Looking at the Void (page 51).

Meditation
Use the mandala to meditate on your pelvic astral centre (*svadisthana chakra*). Examine it closely, looking at all the details. Just let your eyes rest on it, without forming thoughts. Just sit.

Relaxation
Imagine that you are walking on the beach again, but this time feel the sand under your feet, the salt spray on your face and the breeze on your shoulders and legs. Feel everything. You don't have to think about it.

73 The Monkey Pose

Becoming Aware

Assume the Rock (page 16) for today's programme. Yoga teaches purity in a special way. To perform the techniques you need to have a single-minded approach – to be content to spend a few minutes every day doing something that quickly becomes familiar and that, for most of the time, doesn't require special skills. The reward is that the 'uncomplication' you learn in your yoga practice rubs off on your approach to everything you do.

Limbering

Perform Limber 5 (page 11).

Hatha Yoga is the stairway to Raja Yoga.
Hathayoga Pradipika 1:1

Posture

Today's posture is the Monkey (*hanumanasana*) or the Pose of Hanuman, the monkey god. You will need to have at least two blocks nearby for today's posture (see page 20). Begin by assuming the Rock (page 16). Kneel up tall and breathe quietly throughout this pose.

Raise your left knee in front of you, so that both of your lower legs are vertical – the left one out front and the right directly under you. Put one or two blocks under your sitting bones, preferably at an angle of 45 degrees. Reach forwards and down and support yourself on your hands.

Benefits

The ancient reason given for posture work was that it prepares the mind and body for meditation. Poses like the Monkey are superb training for sitting in the meditation postures.

Slide your forward foot forwards and your rear foot backwards, and let your sitting bones rest on the blocks. Stop sliding as soon as your groin stops stretching. Lift up your upper body and rest your hands on your forward thigh. If you feel comfortable, put your hands into the Gesture of Greeting. Stay in the pose if you can and notice that you are starting to do the splits.

To return, lean forwards again so that you can take out the blocks, and settle back into the Rock, maybe going on into the Child (page 66) for complete rest. You may find that you can make progress in the Monkey by turning the blocks flat or even by doing without blocks altogether.

• Precautions

Do not try this pose if you are suffering from an inguinal hernia; instead, perform the Dove (page 96).

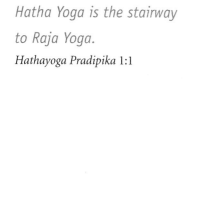

74 A Navel Operation

*The yogi should set aside all longing that
comes from self-seeking, all of it.
He must use his mind to put a stop to the
crowding in of physical sensations.*
Bhagavad Gita 6:24

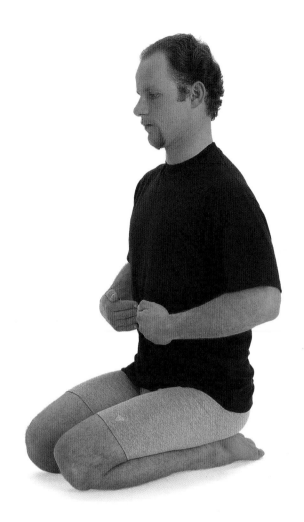

Becoming Aware
Today, try sitting in the Easy Pose
with no blocks at all. If it is difficult,
use just one block or a thin telephone directory or make a note to
perform the Monkey again soon.

Opening Energy Channels
Remain in the Easy Pose with the
Gesture of Contemplation – your
hands in your lap, the right hand
resting in left hand – perform
Candle Gazing (page 37).

Breathing
Today's Energy Breathing is the
Cooling Breath, which will be
familiar to you from page 105.

Directing Inner Energy
To fix your astral energy in your
upper body, perform the Seal of
Shiva (page 53).

Meditation
Take your awareness to your navel
astral centre, the Jewelled City. Feel
its physical position on your body.
Recall its traditional name –
manipura chakra – and say it in
your mind. Become aware of its
function as the centre of your feelings. Imagine you have a golden
jewel in your navel. Now just rest
content and enjoy.

Relaxation
Imagine you are going for a walk
on the beach. Taste the brine on the
breeze as the wind blows off the sea
and then recall the 'feel' of the
beach and the 'sound' of the beach,
but without thinking about it!

75 Serenity

Becoming Aware

Try the Easy Pose again, without blocks, with the Gesture of Contemplation.

The third yogic personal standard is serenity (*samtosa*). This is typical of what yoga is and what yoga stands for, and it can be summed up in the feeling we hope you get when you finally sit in meditation and feel good – a kind of elegant satisfaction. Try it now.

Limbering

Perform Limber 3 (page 10).

Posture

Today's posture is an elegant, serene pose that uses all manner of muscles that other poses just cannot reach. Even if you can't get very far, try the Head Lying on the Knee (*parivritta janusirsasana*). Begin by assuming the Pole (page 17). Lift your legs out until they are as wide as is comfortable. Remember to sit tall while you do this, using your hands on the floor to support your spine, and breathe quietly throughout.

Now move your spine sideways to your left and grasp your left big toe with your left middle finger or place your left hand on your left foot or shin or knee.

If your hand is on your knee, lift your right arm up and over your body to lie on the side of your head. Otherwise, lay your left elbow on the mat, on the inside of your left knee, and curl your torso round and down, to lie on your leg, with your head lying on, or near, your knee.

Finally, raise your right arm up and over your head, so that you can grasp the left big toe with your right middle finger – or somewhere near it. Can you stay in the pose long enough for benefits to begin to take effect?

To return to the Pole, reverse all the movements carefully, and rest in a wide-legged Pole, before preparing to repeat the exercise on the other side.

Relaxation

Relax in a pose of your own choice – you deserve it!

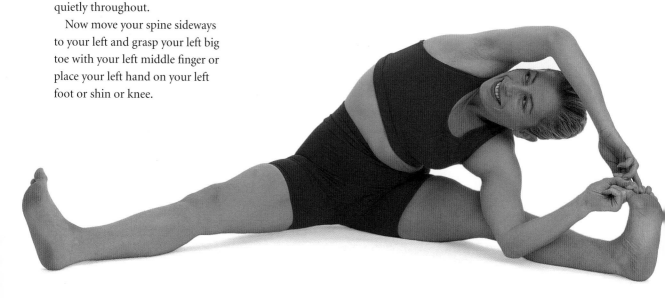

76 Return to Spring

When the fire of the spirit is kindled
When the breath is working with it
When you are drunk with devotion
then your mind will truly awaken.

Svetasvatara Upanishad I.II.6

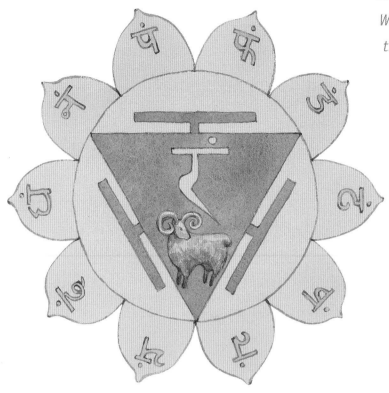

Manipura Chakra:
the Navel or Solar Plexus Inner Energy Centre

Becoming Aware
Today try sitting in the Pose of the Expert with no blocks and with your hands in the Gesture of Greeting.

Opening Energy Channels
Set your astral energy in motion with Head-furrow Cleansing (page 39).

Breathing
Breathe life into your soul by performing the Cooling Breath (page 105).

Directing Inner Energy
Listen to your inner sounds as you perform the Seal of the Six Openings (page 55).

Meditation
Use the mandala to meditate on your navel astral centre (*manipura chakra*). Examine it closely, looking at all the details. Let your eyes rest on it, without forming thoughts. Just sit.

Relaxation
Make a nostalgic return to spring by imagining that you are taking the walk you enjoyed in the Big Poker programme (page 59).

77 The Plough

Becoming Aware

Why not have an extended series of looks at the Half Lotus (page 63). Try it on both sides, and use your best side to progress from two blocks to one and from one to none. Spend a little time feeling comfortable and, above all, serene.

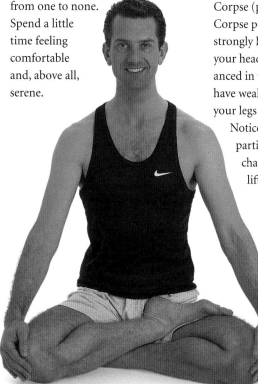

Limbering

Perform Limber 10 (page 13).

Posture

To begin today's posture, the Plough (*halasana*), assume the Corpse (page 18). Come to the alert Corpse position, and slowly and strongly lift your legs up and over your head, so that they hang balanced in the air behind you. If you have weak stomach muscles, lift your legs with your knees bent.

Notice as you go over that at a particular point you have to change your muscle power to lift your hips.

If you have the slightest discomfort in your neck, reverse the movement and start again, with a folded blanket under your shoulders to give your head more room.

Don't adjust your shoulder positions -- just let your legs slowly take up their best positions. If you

are supple, see if you can touch the mat with your toes and even move your toes, little by little, further away from you.

Finally, make your legs straight and strong. Your back will be naturally curved – this is not a version of the Shoulder Stand, but a quite different pose. The Plough is a naturally elegant pose, but it does depend on your ability to lift your body up and over, in both directions. Having your knees bent will help. Stay in position, no matter where your legs are.

To return, simply move your body back again. Let your back stay rounded, but bend your knees if your legs feel too heavy for you to control them.

After you have performed this pose you need to move your body in the opposite direction and rest in the new position for about 12 seconds.

Relaxation

Relax in the Corpse, cuddling your knees to help your spine to unravel.

Benefits

Benefits
The pose works by extending your back and compressing your chest. Your inverted torso will change the patterns of your circulation and open your root and pelvic centres.

• Precautions

Do not attempt this if you have to avoid inversions or are pregnant, or have weakness in your back or neck.

✳ Adaptations

The Fish (page 100) is a good alternative programme.

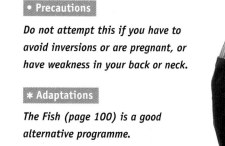

78 Heart Throb

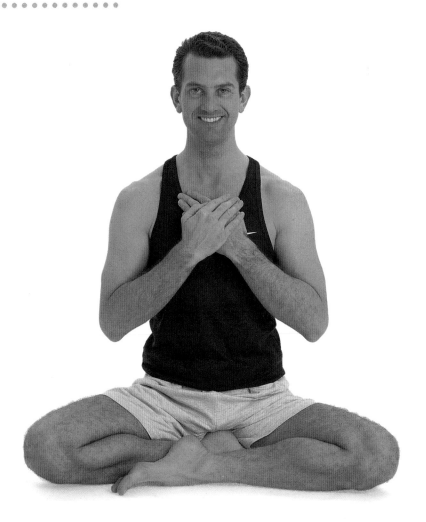

Becoming Aware
Assume the Mountain (page 15), and see if you can stand serenely.

Opening Energy Channels
Remain in the Mountain for the dynamic version of the Giant Leap (page 103). Spend time perfecting this technique, in preparation for Churning (page 113). Stand really tall before you start and step out as widely as you can and still feel comfortable. Place your hands on your thighs so that you can use their support to the full.

If you feel fit and don't have health problems that prevent you from doing this technique, make a strong exhalation as you draw your abdomen back and up. Stay exhaled as you make 12 movements, only inhaling after you have released your abdomen. Exhale as you stand up, and inhale to resume a tall wide-stride Mountain. Perform again if you feel able.

Breathing
Sit in the Pole (page 17) and perform the Cooling Breath (page 105).

Directing Inner Energy
You are already in the Pole, so perform the Great Seal (page 57).

Meditation
Take your awareness to your heart centre with its little second centre, the wishing or kalpa tree. Feel its physical position in your body. Recall its traditional name – *anahata chakra* – and become aware of its function as the heart of your love and the hideaway of your secret wishes.

Imagine you have a jade pendant on your chest. Now sit contentedly.

Relaxation
Make a nostalgic return to summer by imagining that you are retracing the walk you took in the Dawn Horse programme (page 61).

79 The Rolling Bow

Becoming Aware

Try the Half Lotus again (page 63). You will find it helpful to lean a little way back on one hand or even on both hands. The pose will probably slip into place, and you can then explore the idea of gradually sitting up straight, while you are in the pose. Lean back again to release it.

Another yogic personal standard, austerity (*tapas*), suggests a simple lifestyle, devoid of those little pleasures we all hold dear. In fact, in yoga terms it means being really committed to your yoga practice and being prepared to make some sacrifices to keep it up.

Limbering

Perform Limber 9 (page 13).

Posture

Make sure you have plenty of space to perform today's posture, which is the Rolling Bow (*parivritta dhanurasana*). Only attempt this if you can manage the regular version of the Bow (page 102) without the scarf. Begin by assuming the Prone Corpse (page 19). Put your arms beside you, palms up, and bend your lower legs up, so that you can grasp your ankles with your hands. Only pull on your legs to help you lift your shoulders and upper legs a little off the floor.

Then pull yourself, in the pose, over to one side. Roll the Bow over until you are lying in the pose, but on your side.

Rest in the pose and then roll yourself back to where you started from. If you like, you can come right out of the pose and rest in the Prone Corpse. But then do it all again on the other side.

When you have rolled back after performing the Rolling Bow, pull up into the full regular position before finally coming down.

You can combine the regular version of the Bow with this, by performing the regular version and going on to this from the point where you are coming out of the pose and have your legs gently held.

Relaxation

Relax in the Prone Corpse.

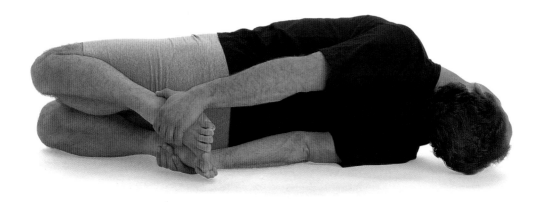

• Precautions

This pose is not suitable for people who must not squash their abdomens or put too much tension on their backs. The rolling over is quite energetic and you may welcome this, but don't be tempted if you really must not over-exert yourself.

✳ Adaptations

A slightly less demanding programme is the Locust (page 92), while a complete alternative would be the Child (page 66).

80 Churning

· · · · · · · · · · · · · · · · ·

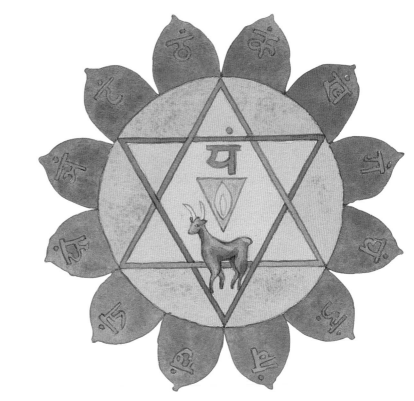

Anahata Chakra:
the Heart Inner Energy Centre

Becoming Aware

Stand in the Mountain (page 15), and make a little vow of commitment: 'I will give this programme my complete and undivided attention.' That's a bit like the meaning of austerity (*tapas*).

Opening Energy Channels

Remain in the Mountain pose for Churning (*nauli*), which is the ultimate in abdominal stimulation. You should attempt to do this only if you can already do the Twelve Giant Leaps. Can you arrange things so that you can actually see your navel?

Perform the first version of the Giant Leap (page 83) and observe your midriff as you hold your abdomen back and up. With your lungs empty, see if you can release the central band of muscle that runs down past your navel, while still keeping the two sides back. Rest and prepare for another attempt. You are only allowed two attempts per programme, but Churning does return twice more in our programmes (pages 113 and 123).

Just for now, perform the technique again, looking to see if you can make that abdominal muscle stand proud, while the rest of your abdomen stays drawn back. Only hold until you need to breathe in, and do remember to release your muscles before you breathe to avoid catching your breath.

Breathing

Sit in a favourite pose for your last rounds of the Cooling Breath (page 105).

Directing Inner Energy

Maintain your pose if you wish, and perform a round of the Big Poker (page 59).

Meditation

Use the mandala to meditate on your heart centre (*anahata chakra*). Examine it closely, looking at all the details. Just let your eyes rest on it, without forming thoughts. Just sit.

Relaxation

Imagine that you are making a nostalgic return to autumn and repeating the walk you enjoyed in the Lotus programme (page 63).

> ✳ **Adaptations**
>
> *A good alternative to Churning would be Cleansing with Internal Fire (page 43).*

113

81 Kissing your Knee

Benefits
In this pose you are rotating and bending forwards at the same time, bringing many more muscles into play than you would otherwise, and you are compressing as many as you are extending. Altogether, a real opener.

Becoming Aware
Today you should complete a third session with the Half Lotus (page 63). Think again about austerity (*tapas*), the third of the yogic personal standards. The word *tapas* actually means heat or warmth and conveys the notion of enthusiasm.

Limbering
Perform Limber 1 (page 9).

Posture
You need a supple spine to succeed fully with today's pose, Kissing your Knee (*parsvottanasana*), although it is one that anyone can try. Begin by assuming the Mountain (page 15). Step out to a really wide stride, moving one leg at a time so that you stay central. Turn your left foot out on its heel and your right foot out on its toes. Check that you haven't turned your torso. Take your hands to the Reverse Gesture of Greeting but between your shoulder blades (see page 45).

Inhale. As you exhale, turn fully towards the front knee, which means turning more than 90 degrees. Inhale deeply and lean back, so that your spine is really flat.

Exhale and bend forwards – that is, lunge, with your chest open and your back flat – until your lips come down near your knee. Gently inhale. As you exhale, make your abdomen small so that you can go on folding down and perhaps even touch your knee with your mouth. Rest in the pose, breathing quietly.

To return, perform all the movements in reverse. Do remember to come up with your chest forwards and open and with your back flat, and to go on into the slightly leaning back position, before straightening from the waist up.

Leave your hands in position and turn your feet to the front, rear foot first, before starting to perform on the other side.

Relaxation
Relax in the Child (page 66).

✳ Adaptations

A simple pose, which works in the same areas but to a lesser degree, is the Moon (page 34).

82 The Bellows

Becoming Aware
Assume the Rock (page 16) for the first three parts of today's programme.

Opening Energy Channels
Stay in the Rock for Alternate Nostril Breathing (page 35).

Breathing
Stay in the Rock for probably the most dynamic of all the energy breaths, the Bellows (*bhastrika pranayama*). We will explore it little by little, building to a full performance on page 121.

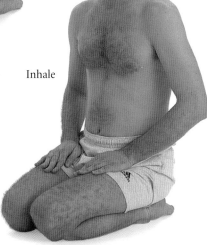

Exhale

Today, arrange it so that you can see your navel. Kneel tall. Look down at your navel and watch it move as you breathe in your abdomen. It should move slightly out as you breathe in and back again as you breathe out. See if you can make only the area just below your navel move out when you breathe in – have a few goes and then rest.

Now see if you can make only the area above your navel move back when you breathe out. This should be easier, because you are used to doing this in Shining Skull (page 41) and in Piercing the Moon (page 85).

Rest again now, so that you don't over-breathe.

Now see if you can perform several rounds of breathing, with the exhalations coming first, above the navel, and the inhalations following, below the navel. Each of these pairs of exhalations and inhalations is one stroke of the Bellows.

Directing Energy Channels
Sit in the Rock, if you can, for the Seal of the Dawn Horse (page 61).

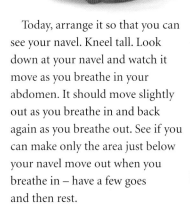

Inhale

Benefits
The Bellows is the strongest of the 'power breaths'. Use it when you need a really strong boost. Otherwise, treat it with great respect.

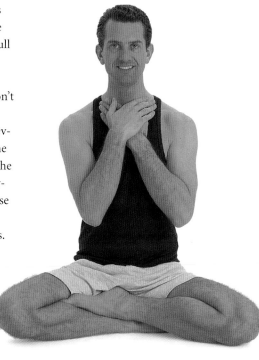

Meditation
Take your awareness to your essentially pure astral centre. Feel its physical position on your body – at your throat. Recall its traditional name – *visuddha chakra* – and become aware of its function as the treasury of your sound. Imagine a soft blue scarf around your neck.

Relaxation
Make a nostalgic return to winter by repeating the walk in the programme Piercing the Sun (page 65).

• Precautions
This programme is not suitable for people who should avoid strong abdominal movements.

* Adaptations
The Champion's Breath (page 45) is a good alternative.

83 The Camel

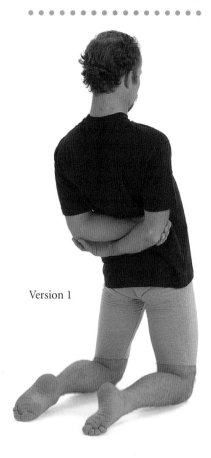

Version 1

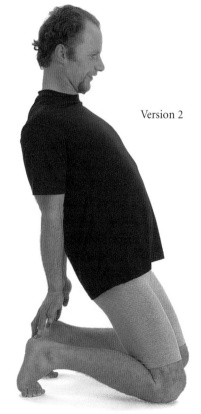

Version 2

Becoming Aware

Try assuming the Hero pose (page 40), for a few moments of calm.

Another yogic personal standard is self-study or getting to know yourself (*svadyaya*). It seems to mean studying by yourself and studying to get to know yourself. In yoga terms, it probably means 'discovering yourself by practising your yoga on your own and observing how you progress'.

Limbering

Perform Limber 2 (page 10).

Posture

Today's pose is the Camel (*usthrasana*). There are several versions of this pose, and this is one that everyone can try. Begin by assuming the Rock (page 16), then kneel up and fold your arms behind you. Inhale. As you exhale, bend back over your arms, keeping your head facing forwards. Don't let your thighs lean back – they must stay vertical, to support you properly. If you let them lean back, you will damage your thigh muscles. Let your head drop back if you wish and if you have a strong neck.

To return, lift your head up first, then your body. Return to the Rock.

A second version also begins with the Rock. Kneel up, tuck your toes under, and reach back to place your palms on your heels. Keep your thighs vertical and your head up. If you have to let yourself lean back, push your thighs back to vertical before completing the pose. As before, the head movement is optional – only if your neck is strong enough to lift your head back up when youreturn.

This method will work best if you have long arms and short thighs.

The success of a third version of the Camel depends on the lengths of your limbs and your torso. Stay in the Rock. It will probably help if you tuck your toes under, but if that's uncomfortable, leave them lying out. Lay your palms on your heels – let your heel-bone sit in the angle between your thumb and first finger. Now push up with your thighs, until they come right up to the vertical position. You are now in pose, with your thighs and hands in position.

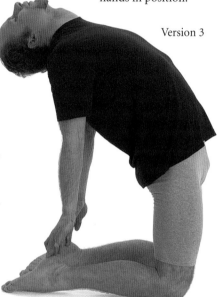

Version 3

Let your head tilt back if you wish and only if you can lift it back up without hurting your neck. Let yourself down again with care.

After you have performed this pose, relax in the Child (page 66).

• Precautions

This pose is not suitable for people with weak backs. There are also several places where you take a lot of weight on your thighs or neck. If this is a problem, you can get similar benefits without working so hard, with the Child (page 66).

84 More Bellows

Becoming Aware
Assume the Rock (page 16) and stay in it until today's Meditation.

Opening Energy Channels
Open your energy channels with Candle Gazing (page 37).

Breathing
Today we are going to do more work on the Bellows. Make sure you have a good view of your navel. On page 115 we explored the special breathing movements. Let's begin by performing a few rounds. Exhale, drawing your abdomen back above your navel. Inhale,

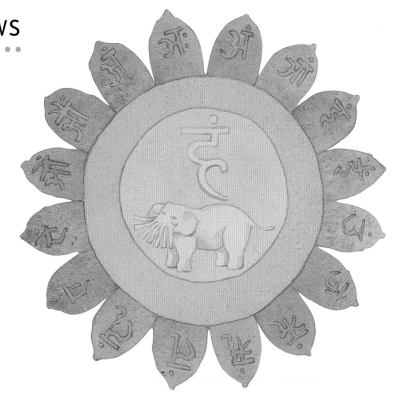

Visuddha Chakra: the Throat Inner Energy Centre

Exhale

Inhale

letting the area below your navel move out a little. Perform about five of these double movements, starting with the exhalation. Rest.

Now we'll go on now to the next step in our look at the whole technique. Inhale deeply. Apply the Root Lock (page 35). Apply the Waterpipe Lock (page 37). Become still and hold the full breath. Release the Waterpipe Lock. Release the Root Lock. Exhale through your right nostril, with the Lock that Flies Up (page 39). Rest with quiet breathing.

Meditation
Use the mandala to meditate on your throat centre (*visuddha chakra*). Examine it closely, looking at all the details. Let your eyes rest on it, without forming thoughts. Then just sit.

Relaxation
Relax slowly, gently flexing and loosening your fingers.

• Precautions
Remember to breathe gently in the Bellows. When you're learning a new technique, it's easy to repeat parts of it too often and overdo things.

85 Three Ploughs

Becoming Aware

Assume the Hero (page 40) again today for a moment of calm. Try to dispense with the blocks.

Think about the idea of self-knowledge (*svadyaya*) and the simple yogic concept that through your practice of hatha and raja yoga, and your kindness to others in bhakti yoga, you can expect to discover that you are supple, strong, calm and kind.

Limbering

Perform Limber 10 (page 13).

Posture

On page 110 we explored the Plough. Today we will look at two extensions of it, but we need to perform the regular version first. From the alert version of the Corpse, swing your legs and hips up and over so that your toes rest on the mat behind you and your legs are straight. If this is a problem, lift your legs with bent knees and only go over as far as your back and your neck will let you. Use a folded blanket under your shoulders if you have any discomfort at all.

Now try the extended versions of the Plough. You should attempt this only if you are comfortable with the regular version. Breathe quietly in the pose and do one of two things.

The first alternative is to open your legs, one after the other, so that you make a wide V shape with them. Check that your legs are straight before settling and breathing quietly. Close them again and rest for a moment. This will extend your hamstrings and open your lowest energy centres.

Alternatively, from the regular position, bend your knees down beside your head, perhaps so that they even touch your ears. This increases the compression of your chest and opens your throat centre. Lift them up again into the regular position, before returning to the Corpse.

After you have performed this pose you need to move your body in the opposite direction and rest in the new position for about 12 seconds.

Relaxation

Relax in the Corpse.

[The Yogi] should set up for himself a firm place to sit in a clean spot – not too high or too low, and cover it with a cloth, or an animal's skin, or grass.

Bhagavad Gita 6:11

• Precautions

We've mentioned putting the folded blanket under your shoulders, but the usual warnings – about compressing your abdomen and having your waist above your head – apply to this pose.

86 The Full Bellows

Benefits
**All the energy breaths (prana-
yamas) are good for asthmatics
and also for anyone who is feeling
low or lethargic.**

Becoming Aware
Assume the Pose of the Expert
with your hands in the Gesture of
Wisdom.

Opening Energy Channels
Open your astral channels with
Head-furrow Cleansing (page 39).

Breathing
Let's put the Bellows (*bhastrika*)
together, without worrying too
much about the finer points. Sit
tall in the Pose of the Expert with
your hands in the Gesture of
Wisdom. Inhale deeply, then make
12 double movements of your
navel – exhaling above the navel,
inhaling below the navel. Let all
that breath come to rest.

Inhale deeply again and apply
the Root Lock (page 35) and
Waterpipe Lock (page 37). Stay
still. Release the Waterpipe Lock,
then the Root Lock. Exhale,
through your right nostril, with the
Lock that Flies Up (page 39).
Release the lock and continue
breathing quietly.

Perform another round while it's
still in your mind – but no more
than that.

Directing Inner Energy
Fix the pranic energy movements
with the Space-walker (page 47).

Meditation
Take your awareness to your command centre. Feel its physical
position on your body – on your
forehead. Recall its traditional
name – *ajna chakra* – and become
aware of its function as the centre
of your thoughts. Imagine that you
have a precious indigo stone resting on your forehead. Now just sit
contentedly and feel yourself
becoming alert and confident –
and able to take charge of your life.

Relaxation
Relax today, slowly and gently
flexing and loosening
your toes.

Bhastrika *readily arouses a special flow of* prana.
Hathayoga Pradipika 2:66

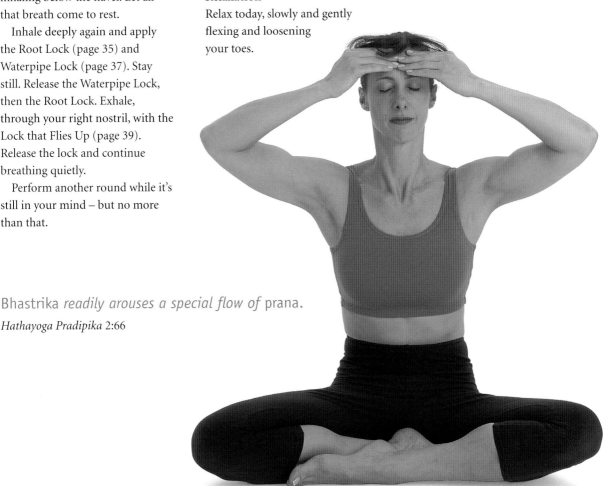

87 The Dog Looking Down

Benefits
Being inverted always has profound effects on your blood circulation. Feel the changing sensation in your head, and your hips. These advanced techniques, with their often surprising effects, will lift you out of a sombre mood, just when you thought that nothing could make you feel better.

Becoming Aware

Sit in the Pose of the Expert with your hands in the Gesture of Contemplation.

The last yogic personal standard is 'offering it all to god' (*isvara pranidhana*). Yoga's origins lie in ancient Indian religions, especially Hinduism and Buddhism, but you don't have to be religious to enjoy it and derive great inner benefits from it. It does help, however, if you can see yoga as an important part of your personal life – more a way of life than a hobby.

Limbering

Perform Limber 7 (page 12).

Posture

Today's posture is the first version of the Dog, the Dog Looking Down (*adho mukha svanasana*). Assume the Prone Corpse (page 19). Put your hands firmly on the mat beside your chest and push yourself up until your tail-bone is way up in the air and your arms and legs are straight.

Complete the pose by flattening your back and bringing your head near the mat, looking back between your legs. To return, reverse all the movements.

After you have performed this pose you need to move your body in the opposite direction and rest in the new position for about 12 seconds.

Relaxation

Relax in the Prone Corpse.

Like a key in a door, the student should use hatha yoga to unlock the door of freedom, by using the power of kundalini shakti *(special flow of inner energy).*
Hathayoga Pradipika 3:105

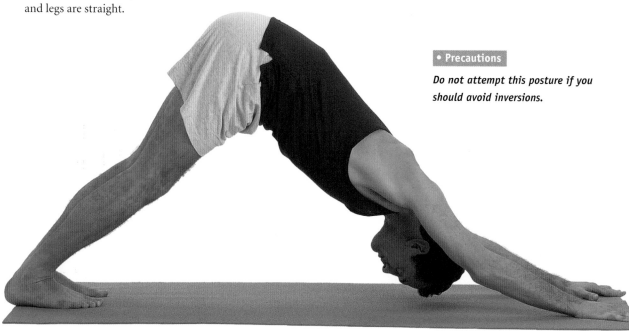

• Precautions

Do not attempt this posture if you should avoid inversions.

88 An Image of Shiva

Becoming Aware
Assume the Pose of the Expert and have your hands in the Gesture of Greeting.

Opening Energy Channels
Today's *kriya* is the dynamic version of the Giant Leap (page 103).

Breathing
Now we will practise a full performance of the Bellows (*bhastrika pranayama*) (page 119). Sit tall in the Pose of the Expert and have your hands in the Gesture of Consciousness with your thumb and first fingertips touching. Fully exhale because you are going to begin with a formalized inhalation.

Inhale deeply for 6 seconds. Perform 12 double movements of your abdomen, at one second each. Fully exhale. Inhale for 6 seconds. Apply the Root Lock. Apply the Waterpipe Lock. Hold your breath with your lungs full for 12 seconds. Release the Waterpipe Lock. Release the Root Lock. Exhale for 8 seconds, with the Lock that Flies Up. Release the lock and breathe quietly. After a rest, perform a complete second round.

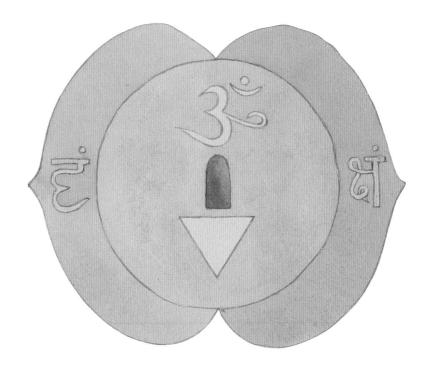

Ajna Chakra: the Brow or Command Inner Energy Centre

If you were careful with the dynamic version of the Giant Leap and quite dynamic with the Bellows, you may well feel exhilarated now, with physical energy or mental and emotional excitement or deep inner joy, which may be a sign that you have a special flow of *prana* in your central astral channel. Whatever the nature of the thrill, let it run and be thankful.

Sit down and perform the Seal of the Container (page 49) to consolidate the energy.

Meditation
Use the mandala to meditate on the command centre on your forehead (*ajna chakra*). Examine it closely, looking at all the details – it is strongly symbolic of the meeting of Shiva, who resides in this *chakra*, and Shakti, who is forever seeking to join him here. Let your eyes just rest on it, and become aware of the aura of Shiva-Shakti. Just sit, quietly attendant upon your own special energy flow.

Relaxation
Relax slowly today, gently raising one knee and letting it fall to the side, then the other and then both.

Real Meditation can only come through confidence, enthusiasm, being aware of what you are doing, letting yourself get carried away, and becoming aware that your new inner understanding – your 'enlightenment' has come to stay.

Patanjali, *Yoga Sutras* 1:20

89 The Dog Looking Up

Benefits
This pose opens all your astral centres, and prepares you for any special flows of *prana* that may occur.

Becoming Aware
Sit in the Half Lotus (page 63) with your hands behind your back in the Reverse Gesture of Greeting. This is a demanding pose, but it's one that will give you real feeling, not so much of calm, as of energy on the brink of flow. Of course, you should only attempt what you can comfortably sustain for a few minutes. However, if you are very supple, you should be attempting the Full Lotus (page 125).

Limbering
Perform Limber 7 (page 12).

Posture
Today's pose is another version of the Dog, this time the Dog Looking Up (*urdhva mukha svanasana*). Begin by assuming the Prone Corpse (page 19). Take your hands to a position beside your chest and turn your toes out, so that you are lying on your toenails. Lift up your upper body, so that you are balanced on your hands and toes, looking at the ceiling. Make sure that you do not let your hips touch the mat. Notice how this posture uses all your strength.

Come down from the legs upwards, so that your chest remains open until the end.

Perform the pose again and try to hold it with still breathing, to allow the benefits to work.

Relaxation
Relax in the Prone Corpse.

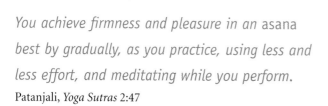

You achieve firmness and pleasure in an asana best by gradually, as you practice, using less and less effort, and meditating while you perform.

Patanjali, *Yoga Sutras* 2:47

90 Roof of the World

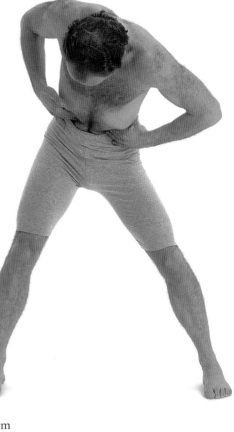

Becoming Aware

Assume the Half Lotus (page 63) with your hands in the Reverse Gesture of Greeting if you can. Release the posture in favour of the Pose of the Expert and the Gesture of Greeting if it starts to become uncomfortable.

Opening Energy Channels

Today's *kriya* is Churning, which we first encountered on page 113. Now we are going to attempt the full technique. Only try this if you can perform the dynamic version of the Giant Leap (page 103) and the first version of Churning.

Assume the Mountain (page 15) and move into the standing pose for Churning. For the full pose, on an exhalation draw your stomach muscles back and up, and then allow the central band of muscle to relax and stand proud.

Lean heavily on your right hand and draw in the right-hand strip of that band of muscle that is standing forwards. It will look as if the muscle band has moved to your left.

Now make the muscle band move to the right.

Then carefully return to the Mountain before performing again. Those movements are the 'churning' motion.

It is quite difficult to achieve a smooth 'churn', and it may help to watch yourself in a mirror.

Breathing

Perform three rounds of the Bellows (page 119), with rests in between. Practising rounds of the Bellows immediately after Churning is a classic method for loosening pelvic *prana*.

To calm down, assume the Lotus if you wish and perform Looking at the Void (page 51).

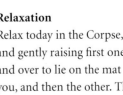

Meditation

Now we go to the roof of the world. Take your awareness to your spirit centre, the lotus of a thousand petals, and feel its physical position on your body, on the crown of your head or just above it.

Recall its traditional name – *sahasrara chakra* – and become aware of its function as the centre of your soul. Now sit contentedly. Feel yourself regaining your sense of your own self-worth and becoming a real person again.

Relaxation

Relax today in the Corpse, slowly and gently raising first one arm, up and over to lie on the mat behind you, and then the other. Then stretch them both away from you and feel thoroughly re-energized.

91 Best Foot Forward

Becoming Aware
Perform the Half Lotus with the Reverse Gesture of Greeting or the Pose of the Expert with the Gesture of Greeting – or whichever posture is just within your reach.

Think for the last time about the yogic personal standards (*niyamas*) and ask yourself if we should strive to achieve all these attitudes before we begin studying yoga? Or is it that we can use our yoga practice times to grow into these new ways of thinking?

Limbering
Perform Limber 1 (page 9).

Posture
Today's posture is a forward-facing pose in which the hand holds the outstretched foot. The Sanskrit name is *utthita hasta padot-tanasana*, and it is a challenging balance, which will make sense if you persevere.

Begin by assuming the Mountain (page 15). Raise your left knee and grasp your left big toe with your left middle finger.

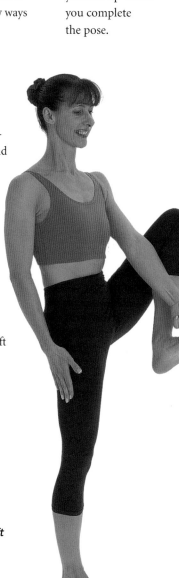

> **⁕ Adaptations**
>
> *An easy alternative to this posture would be knee-lifting. Stand in the Mountain, and lift your knees to your chest, one at a time, taking your two hands to them, to keep them up, while you balance.*

Stand tall and make sure your left leg is directly in front of you and your thigh is horizontal. The great temptation is to reach down to collect the toe and find that you can't stand up again.

Try not to move out of the Mountain. It's better to remain upright than to have to 'pick yourself up' when you complete the pose.

This is a balancing posture, so the emphasis is on remaining motionless in the pose, with quiet breathing.

Perform on the other side, and discover, along the way, that you aren't symmetrical – the second side will be easier (or harder) than the first, but probably not the same. If you stand by a chairback or the mantelpiece you can steady yourself with your spare hand, until you have got the hang of it.

Perform another round, starting with the right side.

Relaxation
Relax in the Corpse.

92 The Full Lotus

Becoming Aware
Assume the Pose of the Expert with your hands in the Gesture of Wisdom. Become calm.

Opening Energy Channels
Remain in the Pose of the Expert and the Gesture of Wisdom for Alternate Nostril Breathing (page 35).

Breathing
Let your breathing become quiet and gradually let yourself begin to perform still breathing (page 95). While you are doing this, see if you can assume the Half Lotus on your best side. Use one or two blocks if it helps. Keep your hands in the Gesture of Wisdom and continue the still breathing while you try to perform this.

The Lotus
Now let's explore the Lotus. If you know already that this is not for you, return to the Pose of the Expert and continue still breathing. Otherwise, take this opportunity to explore new ground. The Lotus and the Half Lotus are the traditional *asanas* for experiencing special flows of *prana*.

Sit in the Pole (page 17) on your blocks. Bend your less supple leg so that you can put that foot up onto your opposite thigh and lean back slightly to allow the leg and foot plenty of room. When it's in place, or nearly there, sit back up straight. This will tell you how successful that first movement is. Stop if it's really uncomfortable.

If you are prepared to go on to try the complete pose, gently bend the other leg and put its foot up onto your remaining thigh. Lean back to give everything more room and keep on leaning while you assess how successful you have been. If all is well, sit back up and sit tall. Remain in the pose to become aware again of your still breathing.

Hold the pose if it's comfortable with your hands in the Gesture of Greeting. To strengthen the effect of the *prana* you have released, perform the Seal of Shiva (page 53), and notice how this takes your awareness to the command centre (*ajna chakra*), where Shiva is traditionally thought to reside.

Benefits
Remember that *sahasrara chakra* works at the level of spiritual being, so your experience of it will be refined, deeply within you, and perhaps not really noticeable at other levels of your mind, emotions or physical sensations.

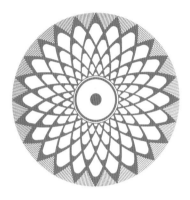

Sahasrara Chakra:
the Crown Inner Energy Centre

Meditation
Use the mandala to meditate on the thousand-petalled lotus centre at the crown of your head (*sahasrara chakra*). This mandala shows the thousand petals, arranged like a cloche hat, and seen from above. Let your eyes rest on the thousand petals and become enveloped in the aura of your own soul.

Relaxation
Relax today by imaging that you are in warm scented water and let the currents give you a beautifully gentle massage.

The Lotus defends you from all illnesses, but only if you perform it with true insight. By its means you will find true knowledge, with the help of Kundalini.
Hathayoga Pradipika 1:44

93 The Head Stand

Becoming Aware

The Lotus with the Gesture of Contemplation is probably the most distinguished of the seated meditation poses, but you should choose the posture that takes you just to the boundaries of your ability at this time. Yoga is about widening horizons. Feel yourself becoming more aware.

Limbering

Perform Limber 7 (page 12).

Posture

Today's posture, the Head Stand (*sirsasana*), is traditionally believed to be the most serene of all the classical poses. Before you begin, note the precautions and alternatives below. It may help if your mat is doubled over.

Begin by assuming the Rock (page 16). Lean forwards and place your arms on the mat in front of you, in a triangle. Place your head in the triangle and lift (or kick) your legs up until they come to a vertical position above your head.

You could practise against a wall or in a corner where two walls meet to give your feet a feeling of where they should be. Now you need to balance, so move ever so slightly, until you can remain in pose.

You do need to learn how to fall down softly, in case you topple over. Try to lower your legs in a controlled way – you will be able to do this eventually. Continue to kneel forwards until you feel calm again.

After you have performed this pose you need to move your body in the opposite direction and rest in the new position for about 12 seconds.

Relaxation

Relax in the Prone Corpse.

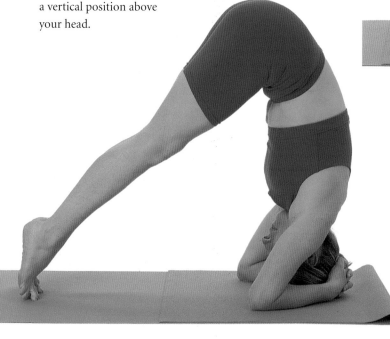

• Precautions

Unless you are already familiar with the Head Stand, you should not perform it on your own. It is a sophisticated balance, and it's better for you to have an experienced person beside you when you practise it.

✳ Adaptations

A good alternative is the Supported Shoulder Stand (page 70). If you have problems with inversions, the Child (page 66) or the Fish (page 100) will be better for you.

94 Four Energies

Becoming Aware
Assume the Lotus (page 125) with the Gesture of Contemplation or any meditation posture that is just within your ability.

Opening Energy Channels
Stay in pose for Candle Gazing (page 37).

Breathing
Stay in pose for still breathing (page 95). In yoga, more is less, so as you progress in ability, so your practice should increase in depth. You should be aiming to do less and less, but to do it better and better. Performing still breathing in the Lotus with the Gesture of Contemplation will be extremely good practice.

Directing Inner Energy
Change your pose if you wish, so that you can maintain it without distraction. Become aware of your inner self, and its sound, with the Seal of the Six Openings (page 55).

Meditation
Meditate on the *prana* flows in your astral body. We use the word *prana* as a general term, but it's actually only one of many energy currents (*vayus*), although it tends to be the most important. There are four main *vayus* – *prana vayu* works in your upper body, your head and throat; *apana vayu* works in your lower body, especially your lowest physical organs; *samana vayu* works in your middle body, your abdomen; and *vyana vayu* works in your chest, especially your heart and lungs. There's also *udana vayu*, which is believed to work especially when you come to the end of your physical life.

Now see if you can stop being so specific, and just feel the energy currents breathing their way all around you.

Relaxation
Imagine you are floating in currents of scented water.

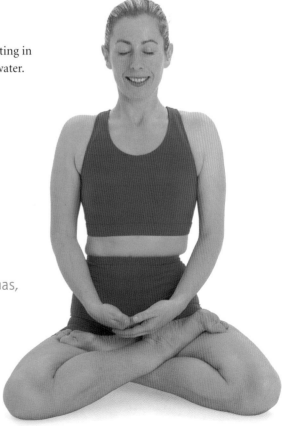

Those who understand how prana *is made,*
And how it enters the body and becomes five pranas,
To serve the Soul,
Will never die: never, never.
Prasna Upanishad 1:III:12

95 The Wheel

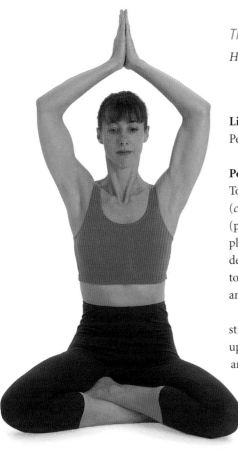

The climax of yoga is hearing the nada *– your inner sound.*
Hathayoga Pradipika 1:56

Limbering
Perform Limber 8 (page 12).

Posture
Today's posture is the Wheel (*chakrasana*). Assume the Corpse (page 18). From an alert Corpse, place your hands under your shoulders, with the fingers pointing towards your feet. Raise your knees and place your feet wide apart.

Inhale. On the exhalation, push strongly towards your feet and also upwards. If you have strong arms and shoulders, you will find that your body will lift up into an arch. If the lift is tiring, you can pause and make the final ascent on a new exhalation.

In the complete pose, your head should be well clear of the floor and your legs firm. Try to hold the pose for a few moments.

To return, let your body down carefully, lifting your head out to the rear as you come down, and settling back into the Corpse.

Decide if you want to perform the Wheel again or if you would prefer to do a counterpose.

If you don't do a counterpose, remember that you need to move your body in the opposite direction and rest in the new position for about 12 seconds.

Relaxation
Relax in the Corpse.

Becoming Aware
Choose a favourite seated meditation posture, but for an extra level of awareness, put your hands in the Gesture of Greeting on your crown inner energy centre (*sahasrara chakra*) – that is, on the crown of your head. Open your elbows wide to each side of your head. This will open the inner energy of the heart and throat, stimulating emotion and thought.

• Precautions

This posture requires strong legs and shoulders. You will discover in the first couple of steps if it's for you; if it is not, perform the Bridge (page 80) instead.

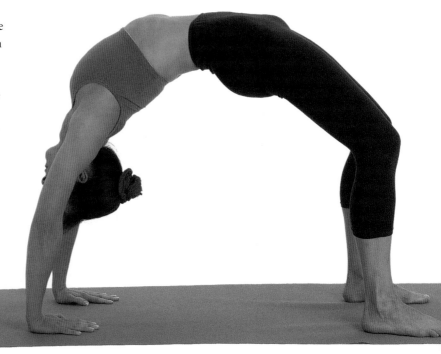

96 Inner Sounds

No altar-fires for me, no wood for sacrifices,
the fire I light is right inside myself,
Burning bright and warm.
My life is my sacrifice,
My heart is the altar,
For I am a disciple of the Buddha,
the fire is my own true self, my servant.

From the *Samyutta Nikaya*

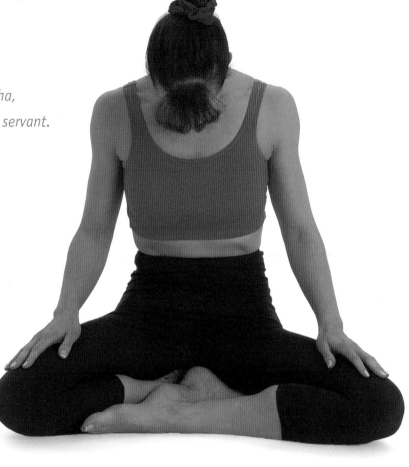

Becoming Aware
Sit in the Pose of the Expert with your hands in the Gesture of Greeting, on the crown of your head (as you did on page 95). As you perform, inhale, lift your chest and widen your shoulders, feeling your arms moving back. On the exhalation, leave your chest, shoulders and arms in place, ready to move them all a bit further with the next inhalation. You can continue with this for a few more moments.

Opening Energy Channels
Release the pose and sit for a moment in Submission – your spine leaning forwards, your shoulders curved forwards and your head bowed. Then sit tall for Head-furrow Cleansing (page 39).

Breathing
Stay sitting tall, or move into the Lotus with the Gesture of Contemplation for still breathing (page 95).

Directing Inner Energy
Change to the Pole (page 17) for the Great Seal (page 57).

Meditation
Sit quietly in a pose of your choice and 'listen' for the sounds of the energy currents, the *vayus* – *prana vayu* in your head, *apana vayu* in your pelvis, *samana vayu* in your abdomen and *vyana vayu* in your chest.

Relaxation
Imagine that you are taking an astral journey and see the sun rise over Mount Kailasa in Tibet, the home of Shiva. Visualize the brightening sky and the ice-whiteness of the snow and feel the utter peace of it all.

97 Lying on your Side

Becoming Aware
Start in the relaxed pose of Submission (page 129) then gradually move up and up into a tall pose of your choice. Then even more slowly, move back again to Submission.

Do all this again, but inhale as you sit tall and exhale as you relax. Think, with real pleasure, how mature your yoga is now – and begin to accept that you are a *siddha*, an expert.

Limbering
Perform Limber 5 (page 11).

Posture
For today's posture, Lifting the Spine (*meru akarshanasana*), assume the Prone Corpse (page 19). Turn onto your right side and make sure that you are really balancing on your hip. You may want to get a blanket to lie on, especially if your hip bones are near the surface.

Prop your shoulder on your right elbow, and when you are settled lay your left arm along your upper leg. Look straight ahead, with your head upright.

Put your left leg back on top and lie right down, with your head lying on your right arm. Repeat all the leg movements from there.

Turn onto your abdomen to rest, and then do it all again on the other side. Repeat for a second round.

Relaxation
Relax in the Prone Corpse.

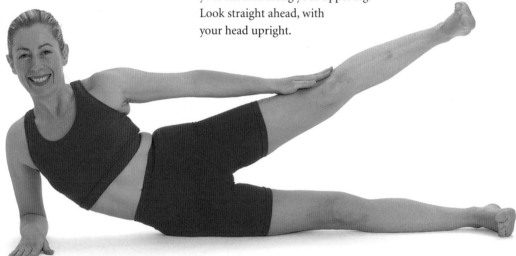

As you inhale, raise your left leg. Hold the pose and your breath, then exhale and lower your leg.

Put your left foot over your right leg and next to the knee. Raise and lower your right leg, with breathing as before.

98 Sunrise on the Ganges

When your yoga brings your thoughts to a stillness and tranquillity, then you can really see your inner self, deep down: a state of consciousness very near to bliss.
Bhagavad Gita 6:20

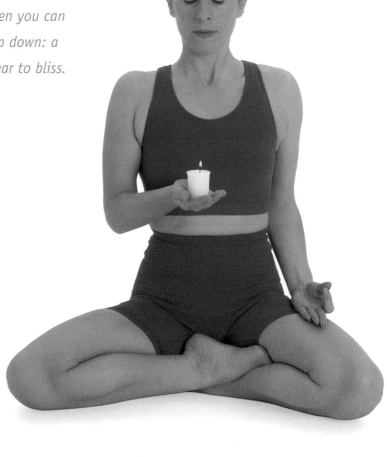

Becoming Aware
Stand slightly astride, and become calm. Perform the Complete Yoga Breath (page 35).

Opening Energy Channels
Move easily into the dynamic version of the Giant Leap (page 103).

Breathing
Assume the Lotus with the Gesture of Contemplation (if you cannot comfortably assume the Lotus, try the Pose of the Expert) for still breathing (page 95).

Directing Inner Energy
Perform the Big Poker (page 59). If you find this difficult in the Lotus, try another pose.

Meditation
With all your new skills and mature approach, return today to your meditation candle and simply perform the three stages of meditation. Just sit. You are likely to experience yogic bliss (*samadhi*), but you won't know until you bring your practice to a conclusion – then you will remember.

Relaxation
Imagine that you are on a boat, watching the sunrise on the Ganges. Hear the oars in the water, the chanting of *mantras* and the cries of the mynah birds.

99 The Ultimate Chaise-longue

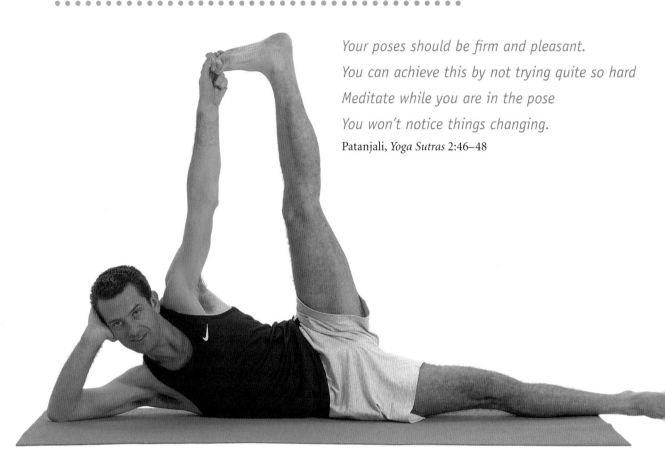

Your poses should be firm and pleasant.
You can achieve this by not trying quite so hard
Meditate while you are in the pose
You won't notice things changing.
Patanjali, *Yoga Sutras* 2:46–48

Becoming Aware
Sit in the posture of Submission (page 129) and slowly sit up into a pose of your choice. Perform the Complete Yoga Breath (page 35) and feel the calmness of all your programmes giving you a kind of serenity that cannot be just of your making.

Limbering
Perform Limber 5 (page 11).

Posture
Today's posture is the Serpent Couch or Vishnu's Couch (*anantasana*), a dynamic leg lift. Begin by assuming the Prone Corpse (page 19). Turn on your right side and prop yourself up on your elbow, with your hand cupping your head.

Bend your left leg and grasp its big toe with your left middle finger. Straighten your leg and arm and, with little inhalations, bring the leg over your head. Your body is a couch and your leg is the head rest, for the god Vishnu to rest on.

Come to a still point in the pose, checking that your leg will allow Vishnu to lie comfortably on it and that you are balanced. This is a powerful extension on your thighs and your groin and a full opening for your two lowest *chakras*.

Carefully release your big toe and lay the leg down. Turn on your abdomen to rest, and perform again on the other side.

Relaxation
Relax in the Prone Corpse.

✳ Adaptations

Lots of people can't reach their big toes in this pose or they fall over as soon as they lift the leg, and some people can't lie on their sides. It's quite acceptable to perform the Cobra (page 82) or the Locust (page 92) instead. If you are among the people who shouldn't lie on their abdomen anyway, try the Fish (page 100) instead.

132

100 Destiny

Becoming Aware
Stand calmly in the Mountain. You have searched for your true inner self – the person you really are – and you can be proud of that and make a resolution to make better acquaintance of your destiny.

Opening Energy Channels
Move confidently into a wide-stepped Mountain posture for the second version of Churning (page 123). Alternatively, perform any *kriya*, standing or sitting, that you can do well.

Breathing
Settle into your most comfortable seated meditation posture for still breathing (page 95).

Directing Inner Energy
Move into the Rock or the Pose of the Expert to perform the Seal of the Dawn Horse (page 61) or any other *mudra* that you really like.

Meditation
Be happy with your meditation candle.

Relaxation
Lie quietly in your favourite relaxation pose and listen to your breath. Think about having your own *mantra*. You've already worked with *shanti* and *om*, so perhaps you might find it good to explore *asananda* (finding joy in postures), *pranananda* (finding joy in *prana*) or *dhyananda* (finding joy in meditation).

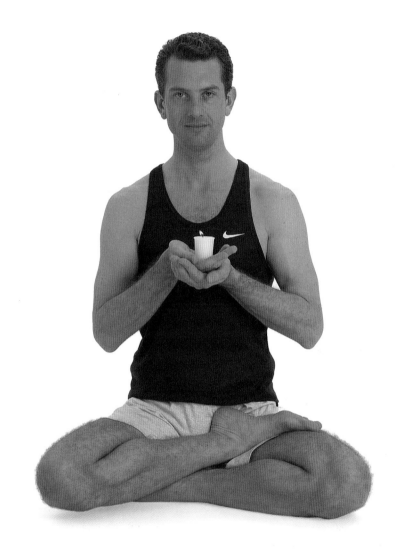

Tat Tvam Asi
(Thou Art That)
Chandogya Upanishad VI: 8

But the most sublime legacy of your adventures in yoga has to be 'Thou art That' – You are the universe, the inner joy, the final self – your destiny. And your destiny is to find that you already are all the things you want to be: kind, truthful, happy, strong and wise and all the other things too.

Part 3

Yoga in your Life

Now you have had the opportunity to try many of the standard yoga techniques for yourself, but you haven't yet had a chance to get familiar with them. It will take time to see how far they meet your own needs or whether you respond well to them.

If you are going to progress with yoga you need to do three things now. First, you need to decide how to make yoga work for you. This means that you must think about how to select techniques and make them fit your particular needs.

Second, begin to build your own series of yoga programmes. These should be tailored to your own particular needs and should reflect your personality.

Finally, embark on further study. Enriching your knowledge will give extra quality to your performance.

On the pages that follow we look at how yoga can benefit your health, how you can begin to build up individual poses into your own programme and how you can go on to learn about and enjoy yoga.

Traditionally, many yoga techniques are thought to 'preserve the yogi from all diseases and death' – and this probably means that healthy exercise is a good stimulant for the body's own natural immune system – especially if it is performed with care and attention to detail. To enjoy yoga to the full and to get the most benefit from it, you need to ask yourself a number of simple questions:

- **What do I want from my yoga?**
- **What do I need from my yoga?**
- **What help can yoga give me for my special problems?**
- **Are there things in yoga that I shouldn't really do?**
- **How should I adapt yoga techniques to suit my ability?**

Before we attempt to offer any answers to these questions, you must remember that we do not presume to be experts on your health. The right person to make decisions about your yoga practice is yourself, and the proper person to advise you about your health is your doctor. What we can do is make some recommendations, that you can follow or not, as you choose. Bear in mind that yoga is intensely personal, and no two students are the same, in any way.

What do I want from my yoga?

You want to enjoy it and you want to feel better for doing it. You can certainly expect to be physically fitter, mentally more alert, emotionally calmer and have a real sense of positive direction in your life.

What do I need from my yoga?

You need a regular daily routine of exercise. You need a daily time for precision breathing and releasing inner energy. You need regular times for learning inner awareness. You need a daily time for formal relaxation.

What help can yoga give me for my special problems?

Yoga is, above all, a life-enhancing enrichment of our daily life, but it can also be a therapy and it offers many benefits.

- If you have problems with your spine, neck, knees or other **bones and joints** the good thing about yoga is that you can vary the amount of movement you make and the speed and dynamic of the movement. See below for advice about things we recommend you certainly should not do and about some ways you can adapt the

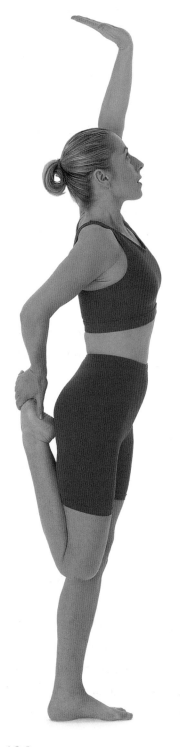

techniques to suit your needs. Of course, you can still enjoy all the other aspects of yoga, and a little movement will keep you in trim.

- Just like bones and joints, **muscles** need to be exercised, no matter how little, and yoga can give you properly structured movements, which will help. You just have to avoid anything excessive.

- Yoga can also help with **heart and circulatory problems**. Precision breathing will improve your circulation and help you to feel refreshed. But do take note of our advice about certain movements and positions. Always read the notes under Precautions and look at the suggestions under Adaptations.

- The general levels of exercise in yoga can help you with some **digestive problems**, although there are important exceptions, and if you are in any doubt, consult a doctor.

- Yoga is particularly good for **breathing problems** because it teaches properly controlled breathing techniques. Nevertheless, it may mask some problems, so if you have asthma do continue using your blow meter.

- The degree of attention you have to give to all of the techniques makes yoga very helpful for **nervous disorders.** Make sure that you have plenty of good and positive things to think about during the periods of meditation and relaxation.

- If you really feel that you are beginning to **'lose your way'** in life, yoga has a wonderful way of restoring your sense of self-worth and it can be useful in giving back personal pride.

Are there things in yoga that I shouldn't really do?

- You should never bring any weight or pressure to bear on any **damaged or weak bones or joints**. This means that you must not bend forwards or backwards without support, and you should not let your head drop back. Do not take any weight on your knees, whether they are flexed or bent. Kneeling may be a problem, as may inverted postures, which carry your body weight on your shoulders.

- **Muscles** are easily damaged and do not repair very quickly. Never jump into a posture. Always know where you are going to before you move. Help a hurt muscle or tendon by 'listening' to it.

- If your **blood pressure** is unduly high or low you must do nothing that will upset the fine balance of your circulation. Avoid having your head below your heart. Also avoid dynamic breathing, which can throw your circulatory system into overdrive. These warnings also apply if your have tinnitus or problems with your inner ear.

- Don't overwork tired **eyes**. Let them close.

- If you have **digestive problems**, you must avoid putting pressure on your stomach. This is especially true if you have either, or both, of the hernias, and if you have a hiatus hernia, you must not position your head below your diaphragm. Avoid powerful movements of your abdominal muscles.

- If **breathing** is a problem, avoid holding your breath for long periods and note that dynamic breathing could irritate your throat or bronchial tubes.

- If you have a **nervous disorder**, or even if you tend to have unwanted and unwelcome thoughts in your mind, always have plenty of positive and pleasant things to think about during your meditation and relaxation times.

- If you are in the later stages of **pregnancy**, avoid things that will put pressure on your stomach and avoid holding your breath. It is also not a good idea to perform inverted postures. Some women also prefer to avoid inversions if they are having a period.

How should I adapt yoga techniques to suit my ability?

Whatever your degree of ability, you should be prepared to modify just about anything, if it suits you. The standard techniques are based on an Indian tradition, with the background of warm weather and a real preference for sitting on cushions rather than chairs. What is important about yoga is that the aim is to enjoy discovering the techniques and not to hurry on to the end of the journey.

We have suggested alternatives whenever we think that a technique might present problems. But it's also a good idea to see how many of the techniques you can perform sitting on an upright chair. You can do a great deal of yoga without getting on a mat at all.

There's a sense in which yoga will tell you what sort of person you are and what you need from your practice. If that means you have to think in terms of years, rather than days, that is a valuable lesson.

Adapt your yoga for the needs of this moment. Tomorrow's moment will be different.
Traditional Yogic teaching

Making your Own Programmes

In these programmes we have introduced you to a great many techniques, but we haven't given you many opportunities to repeat them or work steadily through them until they begin to become really familiar. Yoga works best if you practise regularly, and it is a good idea to get into the habit of performing a selected repertoire until you feel the need for change.

That repertoire needs to be properly balanced, and it needs to take into account the kind of person you are – physically, mentally and emotionally – and practical things like how long you can spare for practice, how often you want to practise, how much space you have and whether you prefer to practise in the morning or evening.

There are several options about your general style of practice. You could repeat all these programmes again, in 10-minute sessions. You could repeat all the programmes again, but in 20-minute pairs. You could devise your own short 10-minute programmes, like these and either perform them separately or build them into 20-minute programmes, or you could do something quite different.

Whatever you decide to do, there are a few simple principles that you should observe:

- **Choose a programme that suits both you and your practical circumstances.**
- **Stay with that programme for a month of daily practices or at least 20 sessions.**
- **Make sure that the content of your programme, and the order of events, is like the programmes here.**
- **Resist the temptation to change the programme unless you really need to.**
- **Keep a record of your practice, noting what you do and when, and the progress you make.**

Perhaps the most important thing about having a pre-planned programme is that you plan it at your leisure, taking into account what you want to do, what you need to do and your everyday circumstances. Then, when you come to perform, the programme is there, ready for you and you don't have to make choices about what to do. It could almost be like a little daily ritual, which you can grow very fond of and which you would miss if you couldn't do it.

If you only have 10 minutes a day to spare, you should seriously consider going through the programmes in this book again, and whenever you have 20 minutes, just put a pair of programmes together – remembering that you can then omit the relaxation at the end of the first programme and the introduction to the second one.

But let's imagine that your circumstances are ideal. Let's say you have 30 minutes to devote to yoga – it may not be 30 minutes every day, but certainly at the weekend and when you are on holiday. In many ways, 30 minutes is a very good time for a programme, because you can include all the techniques in our programmes but still have time to include two or three additional postures (*asanas*) of your own. What would such a programme consist of? We have selected some ideas from the programmes in this book and suggested how you might combine them.

- **Becoming Aware:** Choose maybe two techniques for becoming aware (*pratyahara*) that you can alternate on odd and even dates.
- **Limbering:** Choose two or three sequences to complement the postures (*asanas*) you have chosen.
- **Postures:** Choose a selection that makes a good group of postures (*asanas*) and offers contrast and balance.
- **Opening Energy Channels:** There are nine *kriyas* to choose from. Start with the simpler ones – two again – for odds and evens.
- **Releasing Inner Energy:** Choose two of the simpler exercises, for odds and evens again, from among the suggested breathing exercises (*pranayama*).
- **Directing Inner Energy:** There are 12 *mudras* and *bandhas* in the book. Choose two of them to use with the *kriyas* and *pranayamas*.
- **Meditation:** It would be good to have a group of up to seven meditation programmes (*samyama*) and to rotate them over a week.
- **Relaxation:** Choose a group of quite formal relaxations to balance the *samyamas*.

But you have still only sampled a very few of the techniques in our book. There is, actually, enough material here for many programmes.

One last word: try to choose things that will gradually extend you, physically, mentally, emotionally and, yes, spiritually. See your yoga journey extending out before you and view the prospect with pure delight.

Go on Learning

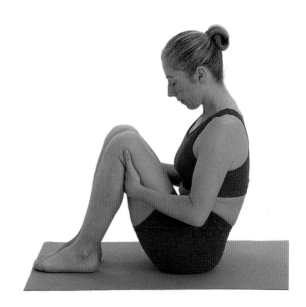

The ideal way for you to continue your studies is to find a personal teacher. You need someone who is fully qualified and has a wealth of experience. Your teacher should be someone who has a special flair for teaching on a one-to-one basis, an easy-going manner and an ability to know your needs – and indeed – to know you better than you know yourself.

Discuss your personal practice with your teacher and ask them to suggest a programme for you. Arrange to visit your teacher, perhaps once a month, to discuss progress and eventually to agree a second programme for you, either to replace the first one or to perform alongside it. This can be an expensive way to learn, but if you only have a lesson every month or every six weeks, it needn't be any more expensive than other method.

The most popular way to learn is to attend a local class. Local education and leisure organizations run classes with well-qualified teachers, and the course content and teaching methods are often monitored as a way of guaranteeing quality coaching and awarding a certificate of proficiency at the end of the course.

Remember that many local classes only run for 20 weeks of the year. So try to find out if a qualified teacher in your area runs an extra class through the summer months.

You can take advantage of the many week-long yoga courses and weekend or day events by subscribing to one of the many yoga journals or by becoming a member of one of the yoga associations (see box on page 141).

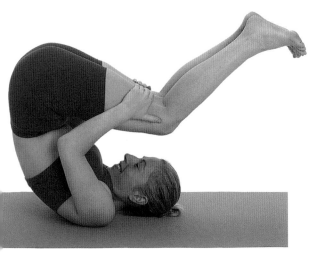
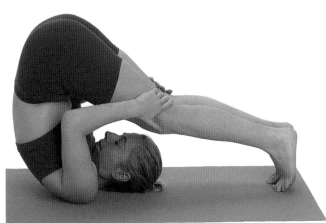

The governing body for yoga in the United Kingdom is:

British Wheel of Yoga
Central Office
1 Hamilton Place
Boston Road
Sleaford
Lincolnshire NG34 7ES
(telephone: 01529 306851)

The Wheel (or BWY) has a network of local representatives, who can give you information about local classes and teachers.

There are lots of things you can do at home. You can, for example, buy or borrow yoga audio tapes. You can use these as sources of additional information – new angles on familiar themes. You might like to use a relaxation tape now and then to see how you react to a new voice. There are lots of audio-tapes and CDs of mood music to use when you practise – but don't use tapes with a noticeable rhythm – it will conflict with the second pulse that you need for your practice (especially the breathing). You can also buy or borrow yoga video tapes and see how other teachers perform the techniques.

There are also plenty of yoga books around. Choose books that feature a particular topic that interests you, especially if it is one that is not much covered in your local classes. You should also look out for the classic literature of yoga, from which there are some quotations throughout this book. You will find copies of all these works in your local library.

If you become really interested in yoga, you may want to get together with a group of friends to hold yoga workshops.

Finally, there are many activities that are popular at the moment – aromatherapy, reflexology, the Alexander Technique and Tai Chi to name but a few – that are complementary to yoga, and you may find that by extending your interest into these areas, you will find new approaches to your yoga.

There is a whole new world out there!

Go out – discover – and enjoy!

Glossary

Adho mukha svanasana The Dog Looking Down (page 120).

Advasana The Prone Corpse (page 19).

Agnisara antar dhauti Cleansing with Internal Fire (page 43), a vigorous way of opening the inner energy channels in the abdomen.

Ahimsa Total harmlessness, the first yogic moral value (page 80).

Ajna chakra The Wheel of Command or the inner energy centre between the eyebrows at the third eye (page 39).

Anahata chakra The Wheel with the Unstruck Sound or the inner energy centre at the heart (page 36).

Anantasana The Serpent Couch or Vishnu's Coach (page 32), a dynamic leg lift.

Anjali mudra The Gesture of Greeting (page 24).

Antar kumbhaka Pausing in a breathing technique with the lungs full (page 41).

Apana vayu A special breath of inner energy that works in the lower body (page 127).

Aparigraha The state of not being greedy, the last yogic moral value (page 96).

Ardha matsyendrasana The Seated Spine Twist (page 60) and the Full Seated Spine Twist (page 68), Matsyendra's Pose.

Ardha padmasana The Half Lotus (page 63).

Asananda Finding joy in postures (page 133).

Asanas Body positions, postures or poses.

Asteya Honesty, the third yogic moral value (page 88).

Asvini mudra The Seal of the Dawn Horse (pages 61 and 79), a way of stimulating inner energy in the pelvis.

Atman The deep inner self (see page 49).

AUM The three letters that make the word *om*, the sound of the universe (pages 85, 91 and 93).

Bahya kumbhaka A breathing technique that involves pausing with the lungs empty (page 41).

Bandha A technique containing a compression, and sometimes a rotation, to 'pressurize' *prana* and stimulate it to work strongly in special areas of our inner ('subtle') being (see pages 37, 39 and 41).

Bhadrasana The Lucky Pose (page 50).

Bhakti yoga The yoga of devotion (pages 45 and 63).

Bhastrika pranayama The Bellows (pages 115, 117 and 121).

Bhramari The Bee Breath (page 75).

Bhujangasana The Cobra (page 82).

Boochari mudra The Seal of the Void (page 51), a way of stimulating inner energy in the eyes, also known as Looking at the Void or Looking at Nothing.

Brahmacarya Self-discipline or god's discipleship, one of the yogic moral values (page 92).

Chakras Centres of inner energy.

Chakrasana The Wheel (page 128).

Chandra bedha Piercing the Moon or the Moon Breath, inhaling through the left nostril (page 85).

Cin mudra or **chin mudra** The Gesture of Consciousness; sometimes also known as the Seal or Sign of Consciousness (page 24).

Dandasana The Pole (page 17), the starting point of seated postures.

Dhanurasana The Bow (page 102).

Dharana Concentration.

Dhyana Contemplation.

Dhyana mudra The Gesture of Contemplation (page 24).

Eka padmasana The One-legged Lotus (page 122).

Gomukhasana The Cow's Face or the Cow's Head (page 86).

Granthi A block.

Guna An aspect of personality – wisdom (*sattva*), passion (*rajas*) or lethargy (*tamas*).

Gyana mudra The Gesture of Knowledge (page 24).

Halasana The Plough (pages 110 and 118).

Hanumanasana The Monkey Pose or the Pose of Hanuman, the Monkey God (page 106).

Hasta mudras Meditation gestures (page 24).

Hatha yoga The yoga of balance, a 'yoke with left and right'.

Isvara pranidhana Making an offering to god, one of the yogic personal stands (page 120).

Jalamdhara bandha The Waterpipe Lock (page 37), the second of the three energy locks, a way of stimulating the flow of inner energy in the upper body.

Janu sirsasana The Head to Knee Pose (page 98).

Jatara parivartanasana Turning the Abdomen Over (pages 52 and 62), a supine rotation.

Jnana mudra The Gesture of Wisdom (page 24).

Kapalabhati Shining Skull, Bright Thoughts or Cleansing the Mind (page 41) is a technique for clearing the mind (see also page 83).

Kapala randhra dhauti Head-furrow Cleansing or Opening the Furrow in the Brow (page 39).

Karma yoga The yoga of action.

Kevala kumbhaka The Silence of the Solitary Breath or the 'still' breathing of meditation (pages 47 and 95).

Khechari mudra The Space-walker or the Space-walking Seal (page 47), a way of stimulating inner energy in the sinuses.

Kriya An action, a way of opening the inner energy channels, of switching on or opening the astral frequencies.

Kumbhakas Breathing techniques involving pauses.

Maha bedha The Big Poker or the Great Piercer (pages 59 and 77), a way of stimulating energy in the base of the spine.

Maha mudra The Great Seal (page 57), a way of stimulating inner energy in the head.

Mandala A design to use in meditation.

Manipura chakra The Wheel in the City of Jewels, the inner energy centre at the navel (see pages 39 and 46).

Mantra A sound with a meaning, used in chanting (pages 87 and 89).

Marjariasana The Cat (page 58).

Matsyasana The Fish (page 100).

Meru akarshanasana Lifting the Spine (page 130).

Mudras Seals, body movements and positions to direct inner energy; also shapes and gestures of the hands.

Mulabandha The Root Lock (page 35), the first of the three energy locks, tightens the muscles of the pelvic floor and strengthens the effects of inner energy (*prana*) in the lower body.

Muladhara chakra The root energy or pranic centre, sometimes known as the 'wheel in the root base', the inner energy centre at the base of the spine.

Nadi A channel of inner energy.
Nadi shodhana Alternate Nostril Breathing (page 35).
Nasikagra mudra Gazing at the tip of the nose (page 71).
Natarajasana The Dancer (pages 74 and 84).
Nauli Churning, a way of opening the inner energy channels in the abdomen (page 113).
Navasana The Boat (page 42).
Nidra Deep yogic rest (pages 59 and 61).
Niralambha sarvangasana The Unsupported Shoulder Stand or the Unsupported All-limbs Pose (page 72).
Niyama A yogic personal standard (page 102).

Padmasana The Lotus (page 63).
Parighasana The Gateway (page 76).
Parivritta dhanurasana The Rolling Bow (page 112).
Parivritta janusirsasana The Head Lying on the Knee or Rotated Head-to-knee Pose (page 108).
Parivritta paschimottanasana The Rotated Seated Forward Bend or Turning the Western Side Around (page 88).
Parivritta trikonasana The Reverse Triangle (page 104).
Parsvottanasana Kissing your Knee or Extending your Side (page 114).
Paschimottanasana The Seated Forward Bend or Extending your Western Side (page 78).
Prana Inner energy, subtle energy, astral energy.
Prana vayu A special breath of inner energy, which works in the upper body.
Pranayama Releasing *prana*, stimulating the flow of inner energy through breathing or precision breathing.
Prasarita padottanasana The Low Forward Bend (page 36).
Pratyahara A state of detachment, collecting your thoughts and settling down to concentrate on your yoga, getting into the mood, becoming focused, becoming tranquil. We have called this becoming aware.
Puraka The inhalation of air and inner energy.

Rajas Passion.
Raja yoga The royal yoga.
Rechaka Breathing out air and inner energy.
Rudra granthi Shiva's Block (page 83), a difficulty in moving awareness from *ajna chakra* to *sahasrara chakra*.

Sahasrara chakra The Wheel of a Thousand Petals or the inner energy centre at the crown of the head.
Sahita kumbhaka Structured breathing as distinct from still breathing (page 95).
Salabhasana The Locust (page 92).
Salambha sarvangasana The Supported Shoulder Stand or the Supported All-limbs Pose (page 70).
Samadhi Yogic bliss.
Samana vayu A special breath of inner energy which works in the abdomen (page 69).
Sambhavi mudra The Seal of Shiva (page 53).
Samtosa Serenity, one of the yogic personal standards, a *niyama* (page 108).
Samyama Meditation (concentration, contemplation and bliss).
San bukhi mudra The Seal of the Six Openings or Gates or the Six Openings Lock (page 55).
Sattva Wisdom; a natural ability to think about life, sort things out and see the best way forward.
Satya Truth, one of the yogic moral values (page 84).
Sauca Purity, simplicity, one of the yogic personal standards (page 104).
Savasana The Corpse (page 18).
Setu bandha The Bridge (page 80)
Shambhavi mudra The Seal of Shiva (page 53), a way to stimulate inner energy in the third eye.
Shanti Peace.
Siddhasana The Pose of the Expert or the Perfect Pose (page 21).
Sirsasana The Head Stand (page 126).
Sitali The Cooling Breath (pages 57 and 105).
Sukhasana The Easy Pose (page 20).
Supta vajrasana The Reclining or Supine Rock (page 38).
Supta virasana The Reclining Hero (page 48).
Surya bedha Piercing the Sun or breathing in through the right nostril (pages 65 and 67).
Surya namaskar The Sun Salutation (pages 28–9).
Sushumna nadi The Gracious Channel of Inner Energy (page 55).
Susukhasana The Child (page 66).
Svadisthana chakra The Sweet Centre of the Intimate Self or the Wheel in the Sweetness of Personal Space – the inner energy centre at the pelvis.
Svadyaya Self-knowledge, one of the yogic personal standards or *niyamas* (page 116).

Tadagi mudra The Seal of the Container or Water Tank (page 49), a way of stimulating inner energy in the abdomen.
Tadasana The Mountain (page 15).
Tamas Lethargy.
Tapas Austerity, a yogic personal standard or *niyama* (page 112).
Tratakam Candle Gazing (page 37), which cleanses the eyes and the mind.

Uddiyana bandha The Lock that Flies Up, the Leaping Lock or the Jumping-up Lock (pages 39 and 69), the third of the three energy locks, a way of opening the inner energy channels in the middle body.
Uddiyana dhauti The Giant or Great Leap or the Cleansing Leap, (pages 83, 85 and 103).
Ujjayi The Champion's Breath (page 45), a classic breathing technique.
Urdvha mukha svanasana The Dog Looking Up (page 122).
Usthrasana The Camel (page 116).
Utkatasana The Powerful Pose, the Raised Pose or Sitting on an Imaginary Chair (page 64).
Uttanasana The Deepest Forward Standing Bend (page 46).
Utthita hasta padottanasana Best Foot Forward, a standing balance, with the foot held in the hand (page 124).
Utthita trikonasana The Forward-facing Triangle (page 94).

Vajrasana The Rock (page 16) is the basis of the kneeling postures.
Vatnyasana The Wind Pose (page 90).
Vayus Special breaths of inner energy (page 127).
Virabhadrasana The First (page 54) and Second (page 56) Warrior or the Pose of Virabadhara.
Virasana The Hero (page 40).
Vishnu granthi The Preserver's Block or Vishnu's Block (page 81).
Visuddha chakra The Wheel of Purity or the inner energy centre at the throat.
Vrksasana The Tree (page 44), a classic standing balance.
Vyana vayu A special breath of inner energy which works in the chest (page 127).

Yama A yogic moral value (pages 80, 84).
Yoga mudra An act of Homage, the Seal of Yoga (pages 45 and 63).

Zen Contemplation; the Japanese way of saying *dhyana*.

Index